Medical Professionalism Best Practices:

Professionalism in a Relentless World

Edited by

Bradley E. Barth, MD, MSLOD
Oluwaferanmi Okanlami, MD, MS
Juan N. Lessing, MD, FACP

2024
Alpha Omega Alpha Honor Medical Society

Dedicated to the members of Alpha Omega Alpha Honor Medical Society and the medical profession.

This monograph is made possible through donations of Alpha Omega Alpha Honor Medical Society members and friends. Donations can be made at https://www.alphaomegaalpha.org/contribution/.

On a personal note, the editors wish to thank the AΩA staff for their immense work and dedication to bring this conference and monograph to fruition. They particularly wish to acknowledge Dee Martinez, who retired this past year after more than a decade of service to AΩA.

ISBN: 979-8-218-51741-0

Table of Contents

Contributors

Bree Andrews, MD, MPH, is the Chief Wellness and Vitality Officer, and Associate Professor of Pediatrics at the University of Chicago. Contact Dr. Andrews at: bandrews@bsd.uchicago.edu.

Bradley E. Barth, MD, MSLOD (AΩA, University of Kansas School of Medicine, 1994) is Executive Director of Alpha Omega Alpha Honor Medical Society, and an Emergency Medicine physician at the University of Kansas School of Medicine. Contact Dr. Barth at: Alpha Omega Alpha, 12635 E. Montview Blvd., Suite 270, Aurora, CO 80045; brad@alphaomegaalpha.org.

Jay Manoj Brahmbhatt, MD, is Clinical Assistant Professor of Medicine, and a Faculty Hospitalist at the University of Washington School of Medicine. Contact Dr. Brahmbhatt at: jaybrahm@uw.edu.

Lynn Buckvar-Keltz, MD, is Associate Professor of Medicine; Director of UME Professionalism Curriculum; and Associate Chair for Professional Development, Department of Medicine, at NYU Grossman School of Medicine. Contact Dr. Buckvar-Keltz at: Lynn.Buckvar-Keltz@nyulangone.org.

Richard L. Byyny, MD, FACP (AΩA, Keck School of Medicine of the University of Southern California, 1964) is Emeritus Executive Director of Alpha Omega Alpha Honor Medical Society, and Editor of *The Pharos.* Contact Dr. Byyny at: Alpha Omega Alpha, 12635 E. Montview Blvd., Suite 270, Aurora, CO 80045; richard@alphaomegaalpha.org.

Olaolua Oladipo Fayanju, MD, MS, FAAFP is Chief Medical Officer for RubiconMD. Contact Dr. Fayanju at: laolu@rubiconmd.com.

Vin Gupta, MD, MPA, is Chief Medical Officer of Amazon Pharmacy; Affiliate Assistant Professor of Health Metrics Sciences at the Institute for Health Metrics and Evaluation at the University of Washington; a medical analyst for MSNBC and NBC News; and a Major in the U.S. Air Force Medical Reserve Corps, serving as the officer in charge of the Critical Care Air Transport Capability at Joint-Base Lewis McChord. Contact Dr. Gupta at: vgupta@uw.edu.

David S. Hatem, MD (AΩA, T.H. Chan School of Medicine at UMass Chan Medical School, 2020, Faculty) is Professor, Internal Medicine, at the UMass Chan Medical School. Contact Dr. Hatem at: David.Hatem@umassmemorial.org.

Eve J. Higginbotham, SM, MD (AΩA, Morehouse School of Medicine, 2008, Faculty), is Professor of Ophthalmology at the Scheie Eye Institute at the University of Pennsylvania; the inaugural Vice Dean for Inclusion, Diversity and Equity at the Perelman School of Medicine at the University of Pennsylvania, and a Senior Fellow at the Leonard Davis Institute for Health Economics. Contact Dr. Higginbotham at: evehigginbotham@gmail.com.

Molly Blackley Jackson, MD (AΩA, University of Washington School of Medicine, 2007, Resident), is Assistant Dean for the Colleges, and Associate Professor of General Internal Medicine at the University of Washington School of Medicine. Contact Dr. Jackson at: blackley@uw.edu.

Juan N. Lessing, MD, FACP (AΩA, University of Colorado School of Medicine, 2019, Faculty) is Associate Professor of Medicine – Hospital Medicine at the University of Colorado School of Medicine. Contact Dr. Lessing at: juan.lessing@cuanschutz.edu.

Oluwaferanmi Okanlami, MD, MS (AΩA, University of Michigan Medical School, 2019, Faculty) is the Director of Student Accessibility and Accommodation Services at the University of Michigan, where he oversees the office of Services for Students with Disabilities, two Testing Accommodation Centers, and the Adaptive Sports & Fitness Program. He is also an Assistant Professor of Family Medicine, Physical Medicine & Rehabilitation, and Urology at Michigan Medicine, and an Adjunct Assistant Professor of Orthopaedic Surgery at David Geffen School of Medicine at UCLA. Contact Dr. Okanlami at Okanlami@umich.edu.

Douglas S. Paauw, MD, MACP (AΩA, University of Michigan, 1983), is Professor of Medicine, Rathman Family Foundation Endowed Chair in Patient-centered Clinical Education, and Clerkship Director for the Department of Medicine at the University of Washington School of Medicine. Dr. Paauw is Co-chair of the AΩA Professionalism Committee and AΩA Chapter Councilor at the University of Washington. Contact Dr. Paauw at: University of Washington School of Medicine, Department of Internal Medicine, Box 356420, 1959 NE Pacific St., Seattle, WA 98195-6420; dpaauw@medicine.washington.edu.

Sheryl A. Pfeil, MD (AΩA, The Ohio State University College of Medicine, 1984) is Professor of Clinical Medicine; and Medical Director, Clinical Skills Education and Assessment Center, The Ohio State University College of Medicine and Wexner Medical Center. Dr. Pfeil is Co-chair of the AΩA Professionalism Committee, and AΩA Chapter Councilor at The Ohio State University College of Medicine. Contact Dr. Pfeil at: The Ohio State University, Division of Gastroenterology, Hepatology, and Nutrition, 395 West 12th Ave., Suite 200, Columbus, OH 43210; Sheryl.pfeil@osumc.edu.

Barbara Porter, MD, MPH (AΩA, Tulane University School of Medicine, 1995) is Associate Professor, Department of Medicine, and Associate Director, Outpatient Experience for the Internal Medicine Residency Program at NYU Grossman School of Medicine. Contact Dr. Porter at: barbara.porter@nyulangone.org.

Antoinette Pusateri, MD (AΩA, The Ohio State University School of Medicine, 2021, Resident) is a PGY-6 in Gastroenterology at The Ohio State University Wexner Medical Center. Contact Dr. Pusateri at: apusater@alumni.nd.edu.

Marie Sandoval, MD (AΩA, University of Wisconsin School of Medicine and Public Health, 1995), is Associate Professor of Medicine, General Internal Medicine and Geriatrics, in the Department of Medicine, and AΩA Chapter Councilor at the University of Vermont Medical Center. Contact Dr. Sandoval at: Marie.Sandoval@uvm.edu.

Hareen Seerha, is a third-year medical student at the University of Washington School of Medicine. Contact Ms. Seerha at: hkseerha@uw.edu.

Steven A. Wartman, MD, PhD, MACP (AΩA, The Johns Hopkins University School of Medicine, 1970), is President Emeritus, Association of Academic Health Centers, and Immediate Past President for the AΩA Board of Directors. Contact Dr. Wartman at: saw96555@gmail.com.

Jenny Wright, MD (AΩA, University of Washington School of Medicine, 2004), is Associate Professor of Medicine, and Associate Director, Medicine Required Clerkship, Outpatient Internal Medicine Clerkship Site Director, University of Washington Medical Center, Roosevelt Clinic. Contact Dr. Wright at: sonic@uw.edu.

Production

Laurie Goss is the Art Director/Graphic Designer at Alpha Omega Alpha Honor Medical Society. Contact Ms. Goss at: 12635 E. Montview Blvd., Suite 270, Aurora, CO 80045; lgoss@alphaomegaalpha.org.

Dee Martinez, former Chief of Staff at Alpha Omega Alpha Honor Medical Society, and former Managing Editor of *The Pharos*.

Chapter 1

Communities of practice: The value of face-to-face communications and in-person learning

Richard L. Byyny, MD, FACP

Professionalism in medicine has been a core value for Alpha Omega Alpha Honor Medical Society (AΩA) since the society's founding in 1902. In fact, demonstrated professionalism is one of the primary criteria for election to membership in AΩA.

The profession of medicine is based on a covenant of trust—a contract we have with patients and society. Medical professionalism represents an interlocking foundational structure among physicians, patients, and society that determines values and responsibilities in the care of the patient.

AΩA was founded in 1902 by William Root, a medical student, who, along with a group of other students, were galled by the absence of professional values, and the lack of professionalism by their fellow medical students and faculty. They wrote, "The mission of AΩA is to encourage high ideals of thought and action in schools and medicine, and to promote the highest ideals in professional practice."[1] They established the AΩA motto as, "Be Worthy to Serve the Suffering," and they defined the mission—educational achievement, professionalism, leadership, teaching, humanism, and community service—as a way to encourage ideals of thought and action in schools of medicine, and to promote that which is the highest in professional practice. They defined the responsibilities of AΩA members—to foster the scientific and philosophical features of the medical profession; to look beyond self to the welfare of the profession and the public; to cultivate social mindedness, as well as individualistic attitudes toward responsibility; to show respect for colleagues, especially for elders and teachers; to foster research; and to always respect the noble profession of medicine and advance it in the public opinion.[1]

They went on to further explain that it is equally a duty to avoid that which is unworthy, including the commercial spirit and all practices not in the welfare of patients, the public, and the profession.[1]

A physician's commitment

The modern era of medicine has brought about incredible advances in science and technology designed to improve the care of patients and population health. At the same time, major social changes are occurring that impact society, patients, physicians, medicine, health care, and medical education. Medical professionalism continues to be a core, but challenged, value at the forefront of all these changes.

A physician's commitment to medical professionalism is one of our profession's most important tenets, and signifies our trustworthiness, accountability, and commitment to patients and society. We must address the role of changes in society, medicine, science, medical education, and the *businessification* of medicine, and other aspects of the modern era with medical professionalism as a core value at the forefront of these changes. Medical professionalism underlies the basis of trust that society places in physicians.

Ongoing changes in technology, changing practice patterns, inadequate time for patients, are affecting the way care is delivered. We must be dedicated to the priority and importance of the doctor-patient relationship while addressing these challenges.

The doctor-patient relationship

The core of the doctor-patient relationship is caring and compassion, and the importance of communication. It is more than understanding the science of medicine and technology in curing disease, it is addressing the emotional and other needs that differ with each patient.

Ensuring that physicians have the needed time to provide compassionate care is being challenged by economic, political, technologic, and financial challenges which also threaten our medical professionalism.

Fundamentally, professionalism is about always doing the right thing! United States Supreme Court Justice Louis Brandeis defined a profession. He wrote, "A profession is an occupation for which the necessary preliminary training is intellectual in character, involving knowledge, and to some extent learning, as distinguished from their skill. A profession is an occupation which is pursued largely for others and not merely for oneself. It is an occupation in which the amount of financial return is not the accepted measure of success."[2]

In 2000, the Royal College of Physicians and Surgeons of Canada stated, "Physicians should deliver the highest quality of care with integrity, honesty, and compassion, and should be committed to the health and well-being of individuals and society through ethical practice, professionally led regulation, and high personal standards of behavior."[3]

And, in 2004, Richard and Sylvia Creuss defined medicine as, "An occupation whose core element is work based upon the mastery of a complex body of knowledge and skills. It is a vocation in which knowledge of some department of science or learning or the practice of an art founded upon it is used in service of others.

Its members are governed by codes of ethics and profess a commitment to competence, integrity and morality, altruism, and the promotion of the public good within their domain. These commitments form the basis of a social contract between a profession and society, which in return grants the profession a monopoly over the use of its knowledge base, the right to considerable autonomy in practice and the privilege of self-regulation. Professions and their members are accountable to those served, and to society."[4]

Professional responsibilities

Throughout medical history, professional organizations have defined a set of professional responsibilities:

- Professional competence;
- Honesty with patients;
- Patient confidentiality;
- Maintaining appropriate relations with patients;
- Improving quality of care;
- Improving access to care;
- Just distribution of finite resources;
- Scientific knowledge; and
- Maintaining trust by managing conflicts of interest.[4]

Since learning requires a clear, straightforward set of expectations combined with learning opportunities, reflection, evaluation, and feedback, the following principles may provide an important basis for medical student and physician learning:

- The care of the patient comes first;
- Do no harm;
- No lying, stealing, or cheating, nor tolerance for those who do;
- Always be true to your word;
- Commit to professional competence and lifelong learning;
- Self-reflection;
- Accepting professional and personal responsibility;
- Using knowledge and skills in the best interest of others;
- Treating everyone humanely, with benevolence, compassion, empathy and consideration;
- Caring for patients in an ethical, responsible, and respectful manner;
- Respecting patients' dignity, privacy, and confidentiality, and their right to make their own decisions about their care;
- Communicating effectively; and
- Listening, understanding, and respecting others' points of view.[4]

Social responsibilities

In addition, there are common social responsibilities and advocacy:

- Commit to, and advocate for, high quality care and improved access to care for all;
- Eliminate conflicts of interest—business, financial, organizational;
- Work collaboratively;
- Ensure responsible management of resources; and
- Advocate for the medically underserved.

Dr. Frances W. Peabody wrote, "One of the essential qualities of the clinician is to be interested in humanity, for the secret of the care of the patient is in caring for the patient."[5]

Physicians must put patients first and subordinate their own interests. They must adhere to high ethical and moral standards based on the Golden Rule - treat others as you would have them do (treat) to you.

Everyone has a unique personal identity that was acquired from early childhood and is formed based on gender, genes, race, ethnicity, family and social experiences, education, communities, language, physical and mental capability, and experiences. Everyone is unique with their own personal identity. For different reasons, and with a unique personal identity, many have aspired to be a physician, with curiosity, grit, perseverance, capability, education, medical school, residency, etc. Over a seven, or more, year period of medical school and post-medical school training and experiences physicians understand and speak the languages of medicine, science, and health care. They have the professional knowledge and experience to be a physician. They have medicine's community of practice, caring for and serving patients and society. They accepted the ethical, moral, and virtuous responsibilities of being in this community of practice as a physician.

Much of what physicians do is dependent on excellent communication, using language and professional knowledge and skills. The power of language creates a version of reality and serves to help make sense of things. Reality is shaped by a subjective view of what happens, which is shaped in language. Truth seeking requires we be maximally mindful of the biases that language and reasoning introduce. Human reasoning and language evolved as a social tool. Language's greatest flaw is that it allows us to say some things that aren't true. When we talk, our words create our versions of reality, whether social or physical.

When I was a new faculty internist at the University of Chicago, I was the head of a new general internal medicine academic division, and I also provided clinical services on the wards and in the clinics. One busy afternoon I looked at my schedule and was somewhat upset because I had been overbooked. At that time, new patient visits were one hour, and follow up visits were 30 minutes.

When I got to the clinic there was a middle-aged woman screaming and ranting and raving about how bad our clinic was, and about her multiple medical problems for which she hadn't been able to get the care she needed. I asked the clinic nurse about the screaming woman, and she replied "She is your first new patient this afternoon, doctor." I thought "oh no," but went in and introduced myself and asked her to tell me about why she was there to see me. I listened attentively and continued taking her history. She continued to shout and rage intermittently, seemingly unrelated to my questions or her symptoms. I asked the nurse to join us for my examination and to change her into an exam gown. I did a thorough examination, listened to her, and found no abnormalities or evidence of disease or injuries. I had her redress and sat with her to explain that I knew she was suffering and feeling angry and bad. I told her that her physical exam was normal. I asked about her family issues, job, and stress, but she said those were not the reason she was angry and suffering.

I was uncertain of the diagnosis, so I explained to the patient that I was sending her to the laboratory to have blood drawn for some screening tests that might explain or guide us in taking care of her.

I wrote her a prescription—I don't remember what I prescribed—and told her to stop at the pharmacy and have the prescription filled, and to follow the instructions on the label. I then scheduled her for a follow-up appointment.

Several months later, I was walking through the hospital lobby and saw her standing in a line for something. I walked up to her, reintroduced myself, and asked how she was doing. She said she was much better. She also told me she didn't have the tests done, and had canceled her follow-up appointment.

I then asked her about how the medicine I prescribed had been. She told me it had given her great relief from her illnesses. I asked her if she needed any refills since it had been quite awhile. She opened her purse explaining that she still had the medication I prescribed.

She then showed me the actual written prescription with my signature, which hadn't been filled.

My hypothesis is this was a therapeutic outcome from caring and interpersonal communication. It represents an n=1, case study in the value of taking the time for face-to-face communication.

Communication

Face-to-face communication continues to be the most meaningful mode of human communication, and represents the gold standard for which other forms of communication are evaluated.

Effective communication skills include verbal communication, active listening, personal connection, trust, compassion, presentation skills, nonverbal communication cues, cultural awareness, learning, education, caring, intimacy, humility, patience, respect, gratitude, emotional support, sympathy, and forming a connection. The human factor is the essence of clinical care, as well as teaching, learning, and life.

Communication can make all the difference when it comes to feeling supported, establishing trust, evaluating judgment, and engaging with others. I understand that heavy workloads, complex and difficult work processes, and disorganized and stressful environment often create barriers. However, effective doctor-patient communication is a central clinical function in building a therapeutic relationship, which is the heart and art of medicine.

A doctor's communication and interpersonal skills are critical to facilitate accurate diagnosis, provide counsel, facilitate therapeutic instructions, and establishing a caring and trusting relationship with patients.

Recommendations to communicate well, even in complex cases and challenging settings, include:

- Be attentive and listen completely and attentively to build rapport and trust, and have meaningful discussions about diagnosis and treatment.
- Always start with an open question giving the person time to talk about what is most important to them.
- Maintain a sense of curiosity about your patient by asking yourself questions like—"I wonder what is going on with this person and their life? Why they are saying it in this way?
- Periodically summarize what the patient is saying and ask the patient if you have correctly understood the key points . Demonstrate that you are listening and care.
- Invite the patient in complex situations to have family or peers with them who may be able to help them to reflect on the issues and explore the options.
- Use simple and concise language without talking down to the patient and recognize that non-verbal communication often conveys a sense of caring and empathy.
- Be mindful of all that may be going on in the patient's life which may affect how you manage their care.
- Involve other medical personnel and nurses to help answer questions when needed.
- Use the right tone and positive non-verbal communication to convey a sense of warmth and empathy to the patient.
- Work to be aware of your patient's situation, and how other issues may be affecting them.
- Be aware of cognitive and non-cognitive biases, acknowledge them if needed, and do not let them affect how you care and communicate with patients so they feel comfortable sharing deeply personal and other issues pertinent to their care.

- Find ways to support your communication with tools and analogies for better understanding.
- Try to keep shared decision-making in mind.
- Be an active listener to evaluate if you need to ask more. Make sure the patient has understood your question or message. Communicate to help decrease anxiety and stress.
- Adopt a freedom to speak out communication style for patients to share ideas with you. Show that you are prepared to listen, and willing to learn.
- Keep accurate records, and frequently share your notes with the patient.

Communicating well with others also brings joy to the workplace, and in personal relationships. I remember seeing and caring for patients in the clinic and gathering in the conference room to complete the patient's chart—we didn't have electronic health records back then.

I would join my colleagues, medical students, residents, and nurses before, between, and after patient visits. If I had made a terrific observation or diagnosis I would share my case with the team. If I had a difficult case, and not sure what to do, I would present the case and discuss it with others for advice and counsel. Sometimes, we would commiserate about the system, or other personal problems. Sometimes, we would plan an outing, family event, or social gathering. This was my community of practice.

Unfortunately, we seem to have lost our joy in being a part of a physicians' community of practice. This may be because limited time and other priorities have limited our abilities, or we haven't worked hard enough to understand and create a social and professional organization within our work communities.

Much of what we refer to as burnout and lack of resilience stems from the inadequate response from our professional communities to challenge and overcome detrimental effects.

We no longer have strong communities of practice.

This is detrimental to medicine, health care, our profession, and us as doctors, educators, and human beings.

Communities of practice

To form a community of practice, identify two or more colleagues, hopefully with some diversity, to meet with and get to know them personally and professionally, and to develop a professional and social relationship. Set up a meeting with them. Learn about them and from them, who are they. What shared passions do you have in common? Do you find joy when interacting with these people?

As a member of a community of practice you can engage in joint activities wherein you can, and will, learn how to improve programs, share best practices, and discuss areas of growth, development, and innovation. These are colleagues with whom you can commiserate without judgement.

Once working together well, communities of practice can always add more members. A community of practice will develop a shared repertoire of resources, including experiences, stories, tools, ways of addressing problems and dealing with difficult issues, and overcoming barriers.

A community of practice is a cohesive and functioning group. It can address unique and important issues within an organization and/or community, and can provide an outlet for social opportunities.

Successful and effective communities of practice include:

- Understanding, evaluating, and sharing unique and important issues in a workplace/organization/community.
- Recruiting and sustaining a diverse team of academic, clinical, professional, policy, and other participants.
- Providing regular forums to identify, translate, and disseminate information.
- Identifying the best strategies and processes for understanding and tackling diverse important challenges.
- Developing an ongoing evaluation of strategies in influencing target audiences.
- Incorporating other points of views and needs.
- Serving unique needs of members of the community of practice

To form a community of practice:

- Identify members;
- Convene and develop agreements about purpose, common goals, expectations, outcomes, and ongoing participation;
- Develop commitments to the community of practice;
- Build relationships and share personal and professional narratives;
- Determine the initial and ongoing projects, needs, and opportunities;
- Understand why, what, how, who, and when questions for the community of practice;
- Identify strategies for ongoing communication and dissemination of information; and
- Schedule professional, social, and other events for members and families to get to know one another and develop professional relationships and camaraderie.

You can develop a useful community of practice with your colleagues, and you must do it. Most important of all, find joy, and celebrate with your community of practice!

References:

1. Byyny RL, Martinez D. 120 years of being worthy to serve the suffering. The Pharos of Alpha Omega Alpha Honor Medical Society. 2022; 85(1): 2-9.
2. Canadian Pharmacists Journal. The Editor Comments: What Makes an Occupation a Profession? Can Pharm J. 1955; 88(10): 7.
3. Choudry MI, Stewart K, Woodhead T. The Royal College of Physician's Quality Improvement Hub – how can it help physicians to improve patient care? Future Hosp J. 2016 Oct; 3(3): 211-6.
4. Cruess SR, Cruess RL. Transforming a Medical Curriculum to Support Professional Identity Formation. In: Medical Professionalism Best Practices: Professionalism in the Modern Era. Alpha Omega Alpha Honor Medical Society. 2017: 15-32.
5. Hurst JW. Dr. Francis Peabody, We Need You. Tex Heart Inst J. 2011; 38(4): 327-9.

Chapter 2

Connection and community in a changing era of medical education

Molly Blackley Jackson, MD; and David S. Hatem, MD

Social connection has been associated with positive mental and physical health outcomes, and an improved ability to cope in challenging times.[1,2] Over the past two decades, changes in technology, generational culture, disruptive social forces and events, and political climate have impacted interpersonal connectedness and sense of community for medical students. These changes bring about opportunities and challenges in how medical schools develop students into physicians.

Several recent trends may have particular influence on experiences of connection and socialization for medical students. Remote and asynchronous learning has been increasingly available, favored, and expected by many medical students; the American Association of Medical Colleges in 2022 reported that at least 25 percent of second-year medical students have "almost never" been attending in-person courses or lectures, since 2017.[3]

Digital social connections (including social media and texting) are now commonly used for relationship building and communication, changing the format and possibilities for connection.

Disruptive societal forces and events have exerted significant strains on the ability to form connections and community. The COVID-19 pandemic profoundly impacted populations globally, and abruptly strained health care systems and providers. As public health responses sought to limit exposure to COVID-19 to essential personnel, medical schools responded by shifting to virtual classes and limiting patient care experiences,[4] which, in turn, made connection and community-building during a uniquely stressful time more challenging.

Coinciding with the COVID pandemic, a series of social and political events have increased division in the United States and worldwide,[5-8] including the murder of George Floyd, Black Lives Matter, the Dobbs vs. Jackson decision affecting abortion access, the Russo-Ukrainian War, protests around the results of the 2020 U.S. Presidential election (including the January 6 insurrection), and the Israel-Hamas war. While these events and forces have strengthened some interpersonal connections by coalescing communities toward equity and the advancement of justice, an environment of isolation and fear has contributed to increased tribalistic thinking.

Changes in health care delivery and climate, including increasingly strained finances, impact of the electronic medical record on patients and health care providers, decreased time with patients, and physicians experiencing burnout and mental health challenges are each likely to disrupt connection and socialization for all health care providers and learners.

Impact on medical student professional identity formation

The development of students' professional identities may be especially impacted by forces that alter connection and community. Professional identity formation (PIF) in medicine is the process by which medical students experience internalization of "the characteristics, values, and norms of the medical profession, resulting in an individual thinking, acting, and feeling like a physician."[9,10] A theoretical model for professional identity formation developed by Cruess and Cruess indicates the central role that socialization plays in the development of personal and professional identities in medical school.

The experience of socialization and the nature of relationships in medical school, including those with role models and mentors, has been evolving. Medical students

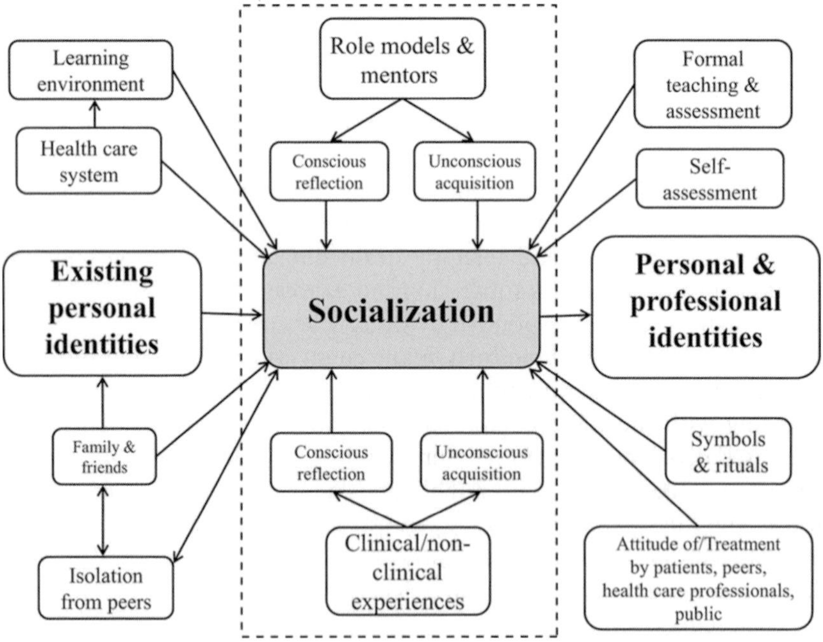

A schematic representation of the multiple factors involved in the process of socialization in medicine in 2015.[10]

increasingly interface digitally (including on social media platforms such as X) with physicians and other health professions mentors, particularly with like-minded individuals in advocacy or special interest spaces and/or with people with whom they share social identity characteristics. Some of these spaces are likely to improve a sense of belonging and authentic connection for students in health professions, especially for those from identity backgrounds that have been historically excluded or underrepresented in medicine. Students also experience more connections with mentors and peers from outside their school of medicine or geographic community, widening the possibilities for connection for many students, and creating the potential for increased cultural understanding and fostering a sense of global connectedness.

On the other hand, the nature of relationships and connections forged in the digital sphere may lack depth, deeper meaning, diversity of perspective, and authenticity. Several studies have shown that the use of digital media for building connections can paradoxically be associated with a sense of isolation and loneliness. In-person clinical and classroom experiences have also changed, as physician mentors may have less time and energy than in years past for teaching and/or supporting the development of students, given the modern health care climate.

The last two decades have also seen a significant shift in experiences during medical school, both within education spaces and in daily life. The COVID-19 pandemic and recent socio-cultural events in particular have had profound impacts on medical students. Studies with U.S. preclerkship students and international studies from Germany and Canada[11-14] during the pandemic demonstrated themes of loss—both the loss of clinical work and the loss of opportunity to build community. Students worried that ongoing restrictions would decrease clinical competency and threaten their professional identity.[14] They also expressed uncertainty about joining and belonging in this new community, noting the tension between the desire to inhabit an identity as a frontline health professional[11] balanced with putting themselves at risk for COVID-19 infection.

Over the past decade, medical students have continued to engage in social and political events that influence the practice of medicine and health outcomes, including in the Dobbs vs. Jackson Supreme Court decision affecting abortion access as well as the Black Lives Matter (BLM) and White Coats for Black Lives movements. Each of these events highlight profound health care disparities for Black and Brown people, and ongoing low enrollment of Black students in medical schools. Medical students have shared reservations about political influence on scientific viewpoints, concern about interference with coherent community-building, and concern about potential effects on their future work as medical professionals.[11,12] The persistence of some of these challenges over decades fosters distrust and disconnection from the profession of medicine for many students, while forging connections and fostering trust with colleagues with whom they share common perspectives.[15]

What can medical schools do to support connection and community?

In the context of a dynamic political, social, and health care education landscape, many medical schools and individuals have implemented successful strategies to maintain and nurture meaningful interpersonal connections among students, faculty, staff and the communities they serve. These include:

- **Create welcoming spaces** designed for both learning and socializing, with programming to utilize the spaces effectively and frequently. Successful MD program learning environments have both physical spaces (well designed spaces that are easy to access and enjoyable, for students and the teams who support them) and intentionally created virtual spaces (to create flexibility for connecting virtually).[16]
- **Assure curricular approaches strongly emphasize group and collaborative work**, including across classes. The 2023 Surgeon General's advisory on the healing effects of connection and community recommended the education sector prioritize cooperative and group projects for learning and peer relationships, and efforts to create environments that nurture mentoring and peer support.[1]
- **Create longitudinal communities for learning and support.** An increasing number of medical schools are using learning communities (LCs) as part of their school structure.[17] LCs are small groups of intentionally and longitudinally connected students and/or faculty who are actively engaged in learning with, and from, each other, often with a focus on doctoring, physician professional identity formation, advising and mentoring, well-being, and inclusivity for medical students and the participating faculty and staff.[18] Using a structure of small groups with established relationships, LCs in medical school are well positioned to enable connection and socialization, and to support students to explore professional identity through space for reflection and dialogue. Other successful approaches include tracked campuses, longitudinally integrated clinical experiences, or any organizational structure where relationships can be built over time for medical students, educators, staff, and the communities in which they are situated.[19]
- **Nurture a sense of belonging.** Many medical students question whether they belong in medical school.[20] Gruppen, et al.'s, suggest that a conceptual model of the learning environment include four domains, each of which have impact on sense of belonging: organizational (culture, rules, practices, and policies); social (interactions and relationships); physical (including physical and material resources); and personal (including professional identity formation and individual growth).[16] The University of Washington Resilience Lab's guidebook, *Well-*

being for Life and Learning, outlines specific practices that leaders and educators can undertake that explicitly welcome and support students.[21] Additional efforts include vertical mentoring programs (especially those supported by staff and funding); robust structures to address concerns in the learning environment and to support students who experience challenges; and efforts to explicitly promote belonging among those underrepresented in medicine (including creating affinity spaces, and recruiting and retaining faculty and staff from diverse backgrounds).[22]

- **Prioritize meaningful experiences in patient care and advocacy.** Despite tightening regulatory requirements, mounting practical challenges, and the recent pandemic public health crisis, many medical schools (and individuals) continue to find ways that medical students can contribute as meaningful members of the patient care team, which enhances their sense of being part of the community. Inviting students from their peripheral participation into a central role in the community of practice allows engagement of learners, and reinforces that they add value and that they matter.[23]
  - During the early phase of the COVID-19 crisis, when most medical schools removed students from clinical clerkships, some quickly mobilized students to participate in administration of vaccines,[24] or other critical service activities. In England, medical students were invited to help with COVID-19 care through specific clinical support roles.[25]
  - Van Eck and colleagues argue for a tighter link between health systems, communities, and health education programs, including by creating opportunities for health education students to participate in efforts to better meet the real needs of patients and communities.[26]
  - Gonzalo and colleagues outline student experiences that add value for health systems and patients, including performing detailed histories to identify social determinants of health and care barriers; students as patient navigators/health coaches; and care transition facilitators.[23]
- **Provide opportunities for reflection and dialogue.** Many medical schools offer both structured and informal opportunities for students to connect with peers, near peers, and mentors, and to engage in reflection within and beyond the formal curriculum. These opportunities have been especially valued by students in the context of the challenging sociopolitical climate and events. Some of these opportunities connect with the arts and humanities to nurture a reflective stance, expand perspectives, and support interpersonal dialogue. A blend of required curricular and opt-in opportunities may be especially effective including:

- Reflective writing and sharing experiences as part of the curriculum, as conducted successfully at the Medical College of Wisconsin for "seminal clinical and personal moments."[27]
- Willingness on the part of school leadership to pause "usual programming" to prioritize processing, sharing, and mutual support during, or after, especially impactful events or experiences, and to proactively prepare faculty who can be skilled facilitators.
- Interprofessional programs using Visual Thinking Strategies (VTS) approach, in which learners experience facilitated art observation and practice deep listening, curiosity, and perspective taking.[28]
- The Good Listening Project, linking listener poets to hold space for health care community members, and providing reflective customized poems based on the conversation (https://www.goodlistening.org/listener).
- The 55 Word Stories project, such as the effort launched early in the COVID-19 pandemic by the University of Washington, to encourage reflective sharing by the broad community of health care team members (https://faculty.uwmedicine.org/55-word-stories/).
- Creating venues for storytelling, sharing meaningful experiences occurring in school and work, through community events like Med Moth or institutional blogs (https://theinterstitium.home.blog/). These may be part of broader institutional medical humanities initiatives for example at NYU Grossman School of Medicine, Division of Medical Humanities, NYU Langone Health, Columbia University Vagelos College of Physicians and Surgeons, Division of Narrative Medicine, Department of Medical Humanities and Ethics, and Medical College of Wisconsin, Center for Bioethics and Medical Humanities.

Recommendations for supporting professional identity formation

With a broadening of who students experience as role models and mentors, and with changes to clinical and non-clinical experiences in the context of a shifting health education landscape, there is particular need for spaces where students can develop their professional identities with intentionality. Students whose MD programs cultivate a reflective stance and create opportunities for them to engage in meaningful conversations about professional identity may develop more complex, embodied understandings of what it means to be a physician, now and into the future.[29]

Curricular efforts in medical schools would likely benefit from an approach that emphasizes that PIF is a socialization process, grounded in community and learning from each other—most medical schools use narrative reflections, which emphasize an individualist approach rather than an approach grounded in socialization.[30] The development of PIF may be especially effective in longitudinal, stable, non-hierarchical small groups, which enable deeper connections, and more authentic sharing and growth, and in groups with diversity of identity and perspective. In addition to these groups, students benefit from connecting meaningfully in longitudinal affinity groups with other students, residents and faculty with shared identity characteristics, and who may share similar challenges or experiences.

These longitudinal communities may be especially helpful facilitating transitions in medical school (e.g., transition to clerkships, residency transitions) as opportunities for anticipatory guidance and mutual support, and during times of challenge or disruption (as experienced by many medical students over the last four plus years). Within, and beyond, these small groups, students' professional identity formation and sense of belonging in the profession can be supported through investment in programming and facilitators that enable courageous conversations (brave spaces), while also prioritizing psychological safety for all group members.[31,32]

In addition to curricular efforts to support PIF, many schools have established coaching programs focused on professional identity. These programs have been reported to promote a sense of group cohesion and belonging within coaches and their small group cohorts.[33]

Conclusion

Significant changes in technology, culture, society, and public health over the last two decades are impacting the experience of socialization for medical students, and are increasing divisions in society and communities. Individual and organizational efforts toward prioritizing relationships and connections in medical schools are needed to enable students, faculty and staff to understand and learn from each other; collaboratively process and engage in the changes in the world around them; intentionally develop their physician identities; and discover both meaning and sustainability as physicians.

The most effective efforts of community-building lead medical students to experience both a sense of belonging and of mattering, with every individual feeling valued, and that they add value.[34] Strong connection and sense of community can help us weather change and create the change that is needed, within ourselves, and in the profession of medicine.

References

1. The Centers for Disease Control. Improving social connectedness. The Power of Connection: How It Can Improve Our Health. https://www.cdc.gov/social-connectedness/improving/index.html#:~:text=Building%20social%20connections%20matters,Longer%2C%20healthier%20life.

2. Boatright D, Nguyen M, Hill K, et al. Development of a Tool to Measure Student Perceptions of Equity and Inclusion in Medical Schools. JAMA Network Open. 2024; 7(2): e240001.

3. American Association of Medical Colleges. Medical School Year Two Questionnaire. 2022. All Schools Summary Report.
4. Lucey CR, Johnston SC. The Transformational Effects of COVID-19 on Medical Education. JAMA. 2020; 324(11): 1033–4.
5. Hounshell B. Measuring America's divide: 'It's gotten worse.' New York Times. July 27, 2022. https://www.nytimes.com/2022/07/27/us/politics/vanderbilt-unity-index.html.
6. Eligon J. Black Lives Matter has grown more powerful and more divided. New York Times. June 4, 2021. https://www.nytimes.com/2021/06/04/us/black-lives-matter.html.
7. Liptak A. Supreme court appears open to upholding Mississippi abortion restriction. New York Times. December 1, 2021. https://www.nytimes.com/live/2021/12/01/us/abortion-mississippi-supreme-court.
8. Remnick D. The devastating new history of the January 6 Insurrection. December 1, 2022. https://www.newyorker.com/news/american-chronicles/the-devastating-new-history-of-the-january-sixth-insurrection.
9. Cruess RL, Cruess SR, Boudreau JD, Snell L, Steinert Y. Reframing medical education to support the development of a professional identity. Acad Med. 2014; 89: 1446–51.
10. Cruess RL, Cruess SR, Boudreau JD, Snell L, Steinert Y. A schematic representation of the professional identity formation and socialization of medical students and residents: a guide for medical educators. Acad Med. 2015; 90(6): 718-25.
11. Henderson RR, Adams CA, Thomas L, Gundersen E, et al. COVID As a Catalyst: A Qualitative Study Of Professional Identity Formation among U.S. Medical Students During COVID-19. Teaching and Learning in Medicine. 2023: 1–12. https://doi.org/10.1080/10401334.2023.2240774.
12. Luman AA et al. Am I even a med-student anymore? A mixed methods study of the impact of initial disruptions caused by the COVID-19 pandemic on medical student Professional identity formation. Medical Science Educator. 2022; 32: 1387-95.
13. Prade A, Keis O, Sebastian T, Öchsner W. Understanding of professionalism among medical students in the first year of the COVID-19 pandemic—a qualitative monocentric study. GMS J Med Educ. 2023 Apr 17; 40(2): Doc23.
14. Williams-Yuen et al. COVID as catalyst: medical student perspectives on professional identity formation during the COVID-19 pandemic. 2022 July 6; 13(3): 13-21.
15. Panahi S, Watson J, Partridge H. Fostering interpersonal trust on social media: physicians' perspectives and experiences, Postgraduate Medical Journal. Volume 92, Issue 1084, February 2016; 92(1084) 70–3, https://doi.org/10.1136/postgradmedj-2015-133270).
16. Gruppen L, Irby DM, Durning SJ, Maggio LA. Conceptualizing Learning Environments in the Health Professions. Acad Med. July 2019. 94(7): 969-94.
17. Smith S, Shochet R, Keeley M, Fleming A, Moynahan K. The Growth of Learning Communities in Undergraduate Medical Education. Acad Med. June 2014. 89(6): 928-33.
18. Shochet R, Fleming A, Wagner J, Colbert-Getz J, Bhutiani M, Moynahan K, Keeley M. Defining Learning Communities in Undergraduate Medical Education: A National Study. J Med Educ Curric Dev. 2019 Mar 24; 6: 2382120519827911. .

19. Hirsh DA, Ogur B, Thibault GE, Cox M. Continuity as an Organizing Principle for Clinical Education Reform. New Eng J Med. 2007; 356: 858-66.
20. Franchi T, Russell-Sewell N. Medical Students and the Impostor Phenomenon: A Coexistence Precipitated and Perpetuated by the Educational Environment? Med Sci Educ. 2022 Dec 9; 33(1): 27-38.
21. University of Washington Resilience Lab. Well-being for Life and Learning. https://Well-being.uw.edu/unit/resilience-lab/.
22. Karasz A, Nemiroff S, Joo P, Blanco I, et al. A Sense of Belonging: Perceptions of the Medical School Learning Environment among URM and Non-URM Students. Teach Learn Med. 2023 Jul 14: 1-11.
23. Gonzalo JD, Dekhtyar M, Hawkins RE, Wolpaw DR. How Can Medical Students Add Value? Identifying Roles, Barriers, and Strategies to Advance the Value of Undergraduate Medical Education to Patient Care and the Health System. Acad Med. 2017 Sep; 92(9): 1294-301.
24. Sinclair T, Bell BI, Perez K, Klyde D, Veith M, Weinstock R, Cassese T, Nosanchuk JD. Rapid Mobilization of Medical Student Volunteers to Administer Vaccines During the COVID-19 Pandemic. J Med Educ Curric Dev. 2022 Jan 11; 9: 23821205211073092.
25. Boggon A, Poole A, Smith S, et al. Medical students as health workers during the COVID-19 pandemic. BMJ Leader. 2023; 7: 149-51.
26. Van Eck RN, Gullett HL, Lamb SM, Krouse HJ, et al. The power of interdependence: Linking health systems, communities, and health professions educational programs to better meet the needs of patients and populations. Medical Teacher. 2021; 43: S32–38.
27. Campbell BH, Treat R, Johnson, B, Derse A. Creating Reflective Space for Reflective and "Unreflective" Medical Students: Exploring Seminal Moments in a Large-Group Writing Session. Acad Med. June 2020. 95(6): 882-7.
28. Paul A, Mercado N, Block L, DeVoe B, et al. Visual thinking strategies for interprofessional education and promoting collaborative competencies. Clin Teach. 2023 Oct; 20(5): e13644.
29. Monrouxe LV, Rees CE, Hu W. Differences in medical students' explicit discourses of professionalism: acting, representing, becoming. Med Educ. 2011 Jun; 45(6): 585-602.
30. Mount GR, Kahlke R, Melton J, Varpio L. A Critical Review of Professional Identity Formation Interventions in Medical Education. Acad Med. 2022 Nov 1; 97(11S): S96-S106.
31. Wasserman JA, Browne BJ. On Triggering and Being Triggered: Civil Society and Building Brave Spaces in Medical Education. Teaching and Learning in Medicine. 2021; 33(5) 561-7.
32. Myers K, Trull LH, Bryson BJ, Yeom HS. Affinity Groups: Redefining Brave Spaces J Baccalaureate Social Work. 2019; 24:1–18.
33. Hauer KE, Chang A, van Schaik SM, Lucey C, et al. It's All About the Trust And Building A Foundation: Evaluation of a Longitudinal Medical Student Coaching Program. Teaching and Learning in Medicine. 2023; 35: 550–64.
34. Prilleltensky I, Dietz S, Zopluoglu C, Clarke A, et al. Assessing a culture of mattering in a higher education context. J Study of Postsecondary and Tertiary Education. 2020; 5: 58-104.

Chapter 3

Professionalism: Yesterday, today, and what comes tomorrow in a relentlessly changing world

Olaoluwa Oladipo Fayanju, MD, MS, FAAFP

The White Coat Ceremony has become such an accepted rite of passage into the medical profession that most new, and most more-seasoned, physicians are unaware that the ceremony is a recent invention. The first White Coat Ceremony took place at the University of Chicago's Pritzker School of Medicine in 1989, but the first official White Coat Ceremony was established under the auspices of the Arnold P. Gold Foundation in 1993 at Columbia University.[1] Back then, Dr. Arnold Gold,[2] a renowned neurologist and beloved physician-teacher known for his charismatic, humanistic, and patient centered-commitment to medicine, had first-year medical students engage in the donning of short white coats and the storied, but far more ancient rite, of medical professionalism: the recitation of the Hippocratic Oath.

Ceremonies and oaths that originated from thousands of years ago may seem out of place in most fields, but they are some of the foundational and demonstrative ways doctors define their profession, demonstrate fidelity to their values, and show their commitment to colleagues and patients. These moments matter because they celebrate the different roads that brought each student to that moment, and because of the symbolism of what lies ahead. The ceremonies and oaths transform the participants and enshrine them in a unique fraternity. One is no longer just a person, but a medical professional imbued with the formidable responsibilities and pressures of conducting oneself in a manner that aligns with values and standards developed over the course of three millennia.

However, for many students, colleagues, and peers, the expectations of the profession are incongruent, vague, and incompatible with modern times. Modern definitions of professionalism, although shaped and formed by medicine's forebearers, are primarily the product of a mostly male and mostly white profession that possesses a world view that does not neatly align with an evolving and increasingly diverse fraternity of clinicians.

The current state

How did we arrive at our current state of medical professionalism, and what does the future hold as we train, teach, learn, and treat patients in an ever-changing world? Like any thorough physician, the factors that now define medical professionalism are:

- Practicing patient-centered care that prioritizes the health and well-being of patients, respecting their dignity and caring for their needs.
- Maintaining an ethical practice that adheres to principles of confidentiality, informed consent, and honesty.
- Fulfilling a social responsibility that recognizes the unique and essential role of physicians lending their voice to issues that worsen disparities, reduce equity or negatively impact public health.
- Cultural competency that demonstrates an understanding and respect of cultural differences to ensure effective communication and high quality care.

Historical evolution of medical professionalism: Hippocrates

The foundation of medical professionalism in ancient Greece is rooted in the teachings of Hippocrates (c 460–370 BCE). Hippocrates, widely known as the Father of Medicine, articulated the key principles that in his time, defined medical ethics and professionalism, and are central to how we define the concept today.

Beneficence

The principle of beneficence mandates actions that promote the well-being of patients and is central to the Hippocratic Oath's directive to "benefit the sick." This principle is not merely about avoiding harm, but actively contributing to the health and welfare of patients, and emphasizing the altruistic foundation of all medical practice.

Non-maleficence

Non-maleficence is commonly understood and interpreted as "First, do no harm" (*Primum non nocere*). Similar to the beneficence principle, it underscores the importance of considering the potential harm of any medical intervention and the ethical obligation to avoid causing harm to patients.

Confidentiality

Confidentiality is another cornerstone of Hippocratic medicine and the clearest connection to concepts of trust in the oath. The oath includes commitments to respect the privacy of patients' lives and conditions, and recognizing the trust placed in physicians by those they treat. Today, the modern concept of patient confidentiality, emphasizing the protection of patient information within the health care setting is one of the more practical day-to-day embodiments of this principle.

Taken together these principles—with their focus on ethics, compassion, and patient care—provide the symbolic and practical underpinnings of an oath that defines the medical profession's commitment to high ethical standards.[3,4,5]

The advent of medical science and medical professionalism: 5th century BCE - 18th century

Across the span of history, between the time of Hippocrates (the 5th century BCE) and the birth of the modern era in medicine, professionalism, while grounded in Hippocratic principles, evolved. After Hippocrates, Galen (129-26 CE), a medical scholar and polymath who wrote on medicine, anatomy, physiology, linguistics and philosophy, was a major influence on successive generations.[6] In medicine, Galen's enduring legacy goes beyond his writings, which would define the art, if not the science, of medicine well into the 17th and 18th centuries. Galen wrote how even with a vast amount of information, the ethical challenge of medical decision-making persists and is made more difficult by the highly variable nature of outcomes, even when best practices are implemented. Galen advocated for an approach to medicine that recognized the limits of human knowledge (and his limited scientific understanding) and aimed to get as close to the ideal of comprehensive understanding as possible. As such, his arguments against purely empirical approaches to medicine were combined with a belief in the need for philosophical observations and theoretical innovation to address novel or uncertain pathological conditions.[7] These were by no means comprehensive or perfect principles (later scholars would refute the lack of evidence and errors in his anatomical conclusions), yet they remain relevant in contemporary medicine and guide professional standards, especially in the face of new diseases like HIV/AIDS in the 1980s and, more recently, COVID-19.

The Middle Ages witnessed the consolidation of Galenic and Hippocratic principles with Islamic scholarship and Christian theology that led to a blend of influences, such as herbal remedies were utilized, and how medical care was provided in monastic settings and early hospitals. Public perceptions of the medical profession came under scrutiny and increased pressure as crises like the Black Death ravaged populations in Europe, Western and Central Asia and North Africa.[8,9] In the face of such catastrophic events, explanations for the pandemic, specifically, and physiological processes in general, turned to the supernatural, with many seeing the plague as divine punishment for sins. These events took the profession backward even as innovations made necessary to combat the plague–more effective quarantine practices, increased attention to sanitation, a nascent public health infrastructure—first emerged.[10]

In the Renaissance (c. 14th—17th centuries), reassessment of old texts and past doctrine further changed the practice and teaching of medicine. Andreas Vesalius (1514–1564) would do work that represented a seismic shift in the medical world, emphasizing empirical observation over reliance on ancient texts which lacked the rigorousness of a more scientific method. As the Scientific Revolution took hold in the 17th century, William Harvey would build on the work of Vesalius as he and his contemporaries introduced empirical methodologies and experimental techniques.[11] Harvey's insistence on empirical evidence, and his methodical approach to disproving Galenic anatomical and physiology conclusions, highlighted the importance of skepticism, inquiry, and the continual testing of hypotheses within medical practice. These principles became integral to the evolving definitions of medical professionalism, emphasizing the need for ongoing learning, adaptation, and the application of scientific methodologies to clinical practice. His work challenged physicians to reconsider their understanding of the human body (he successfully demonstrated the presence of the human circulatory system through extensive dissection of cadavers), hastening a move away from speculative medicine toward a more rigorous, evidence-based practice. This shift necessitated a re-evaluation of the medical profession's role from protectors of what was considered accepted know-how and practice to pioneers of scientific discovery and innovation.

Edward Jenner's discovery of the smallpox vaccine in 1796 was transformative for its approach to disease prevention and for shaping the future of professional medicine. For Jenner and his contemporaries, the practices and educational structures of medicine were already rapidly changing. Divisions between traditionally trained physicians and surgeons, who often gained their medical knowledge through apprenticeship, began to recede and be less distinct.

New teaching hospitals in Europe and in the United States—the first at the University of Pennsylvania, founded in 1765 on the eve of the American Revolution—emerged as centralized, and increasingly respected destinations for learning and collaboration. These new institutions and the introduction of Jenner's vaccine, were landmark achievements for the profession and for the credibility of medical science. This was a pivotal moment that demonstrated, as Harvey had done a century before, the value and importance of scientific innovation in medical practice and professionalism.[12]

Formalizing medical education in the U.S., the rise of the academic medicine and the impacts of the 1910 Flexner Report

The advances of medical education and professionalism witnessed in the U.S. at the end of the colonial era were part of a larger movement in the new nation. In the United Kingdom and in America, doctors sought to create educational and professional institutions like medical schools and medical societies that gave doctors more distinctive and exclusive status.[13] However, at least in the U.S., the influences of the burgeoning democracy would run head first into the inegalitarian desires of the American medical profession.[13]

As Paul Starr described in his seminal work *The Social Transformation of American Medicine,* the most common construct of life in the first century of the U.S.—largely agrarian and self-reliant by necessity in both rural and urban locations—also lent itself to resistance against authority with much of the public "refusing to grant [the medical profession] any privileges" while "asserting their own rights to judgment in managing sickness."[13] Even with advances like the smallpox inoculation, some medical professionals, and the lay public, questioned whether therapies were effective and whether it was wise to keep the knowledge and trust of treatment in the hands of a few.

Three spheres of practice emerged that divided medical care for most of the 19th century: the medicine of the domestic household, the medicine of the physicians, and the medicine of the layhealers.[13] Domestic medicine was practiced in the home and often by members of the family with no training. It was reliant on traditional remedies and basic practices that were passed down from one generation to the next with simple cures and therapies at their foundation. Formal training or instruction was dependent on texts like William Buchan's *Domestic Medicine,* and John C. Gunn's 1830 book of the same name. Lay medicine was also practiced by people without formal medical training but who possessed knowledge and skills. They included midwives, herbalists, and community-based providers who had practical experience. Domestic and lay medicine, unlike physician medicine, was practiced primarily by women, and Black men and women, and was open and accessible to a much larger proportion of the population.

Meanwhile, physician-based medicine grew, and the institutions that defined it—medical schools and medical societies—sought the means to protect, enhance and codify the professional status of the American medical doctor through the authority of medical degrees, credentials, and licensure. Initially honorific, the first law requiring a license for the practice of medicine was issued by New York City in 1760. Following independence from Great Britain, new states extended to medical societies the authority to grant licensure but it had little impact or real power to guarantee the quality or efficacy of practitioners or the care they rendered. No standards were established for medical school curriculum or the duration of training, and because medical societies and medical schools were paid by those seeking either licensure or degree, respectively (with payment withheld by the applicant if they were denied or failed), this system created a perverse incentive that undermined the profession. Also, the rise of medical societies and licensure accelerated, and made permanent, the exclusion of women and all but a relative few minorities from physician medicine for much of the 19th century and well into the 20th century.

As the U.S. continued through the middle decades of the 19th century, an era marked by regional division, the Civil War, and the abolition of slavery resulted in a crisis of credibility in the medical profession that mirrored the tumult that the nation was enduring. The proliferation of medical schools and easy access to degrees, saw the ranks of the American medical profession continue to grow but without standards or unifying institutions. Quackery and fraud was prevalent, which further degraded the reputation of the profession. The founding of the American Medical Association (AMA) in 1847 was a response to the discontent of physicians who saw stagnation in their status and feared further erosion. The AMA sought to raise and standardize, requirements for medical degrees, support scientific advancement in the field, codify medical ethics, and improve public health at a time when licensure standards were being repealed due to the perception that they were ineffectual and anti-democratic.[14] The early AMA had little substantive influence until much later in the 19th century and did so only after overcoming the internal strife that had torn apart the profession for most of the preceding century.[13] Rivalry, and the battle for the legitimate ownership of medical professionalism between the regular allopathic physicians, the growing homeopathic movement, and later osteopathic practitioners, gave way to consolidation of medical societies and ultimately the primacy of the AMA. Concurrently, the reform of medical education, beginning at institutions like Harvard and Johns Hopkins, took form as medical instruction in the U.S. began to reflect what was emerging in Europe where laboratory sciences such as physiology, chemistry, histology, pathology, anatomy, and bacteriology grounded new students in the fundamentals of medical science.

Once it had established its primacy over the American medical profession at the start of the 20th century, the AMA would be instrumental in reforms and changes that would define the next 120 years of graduate medical education. Starting first with the Council of Medical Education in 1904, the AMA established the minimum standards for entry into medical school, and standard curriculum required during the four years of training. In 1906, the AMA categorized all 160 medical schools in the U.S., assigning each to different classes. Class A schools represented what was considered the best most comprehensive institutions; Class B consisted of schools with challenges, but which were deemed redeemable; and Class C schools were considered beyond salvageable.

The results of this analysis were given to an outside group, the Carnegie Foundation, to conduct a follow-up study, and to provide recommendations. Led by Abraham Flexner, the study and the report he published in 1910 had a profound and lasting effect on medical education. Thanks in part to his report, the number of medical schools decreased from a high of 165 in 1906 to 131 by the end of 1910.[15] While multiple factors including the changing economics of licensure fees, and tuition, and rising direct and indirect costs, led many schools to close, the report is credited with improving the quality and consistency of medical education, and imposing stringent admissions criteria.[16]

Less discussed was the impact of the report and the school closures in making American medicine less socially, racially, and economically diverse than it already was. Of the seven predominantly black medical schools that existed before the Flexner report, only two (Howard and Meharry) remained after the report's publication. Flexner's own views on race, and his belief that African-American physicians were not needed beyond the "sanitary" needs of the community contributed to significant setbacks in the training of Black physicians, and reinforced existing inequalities in the U.S. medical and health care system.[17] Taken together, more stringent admissions requirements, the higher cost of educating medical students, the opportunity cost of residency training combined with deliberate policies that discriminated against Blacks, Jews, immigrants, women, and really any person of lower socioeconomic status ensured that the ranks of American medicine were dominated by white men. It was not until the middle of the 20th century that changes spurred by the Civil Rights movement began to reopen the doors of medicine to people of more diverse backgrounds.

Medical professionalism today and tomorrow: New standards for a changing nation

Over the last 50 years, medical professionalism, which had been defined largely by adherence to, and expertise in medical science; its appropriate application in patient care; and ethical standards and practices established by a homogenous social cohort, evolved to reflect the environment we live and work in today. Two contemporary forces have been key to this change.

Diversification of the Clinical Workforce

Efforts to increase diversity in medical schools, and the overall health care workforce, gained momentum during the 1960s through to the present day. This change has been gradual and slower than many would hope but it has persisted thanks to policy changes, scholarships and financial support to underrepresented groups, targeted recruitment, and affirmative action programs that have recognized the lingering impact of past discrimination. Title VI of the Civil Rights Act of 1964 specifically impacted the funding of institutions like medical schools requiring the elimination of discriminatory practices which created opportunities for minorities.

Along with Title VI, affirmative action policies such as Executive Order 11246 in 1965, established requirements that health care institutions including medical schools and hospitals needed to take active steps to increase employment and education opportunities for minorities.[18]

While government has played a key role, medical schools also took organized steps to meet the moment. Since the late 1960s, the Association of American Medical Colleges (AAMC) has emphasized the importance of minority admissions, and has introduced and given support to initiatives and guidelines that promote diversity in medical education.[19] Added to that, the admissions process has changed to consider a wide range of factors which include academic performance and life experience, leadership qualities, and a commitment to service and serving diverse communities. Permanent offices and programs dedicated to diversity, retention, and mentorship of students and faculty has also moved the profession forward.

Progress has been slow, and after nearly five decades of these efforts, there is still room for significant improvement. In 2018, 5.4 percent of physicians were Black in a population that was 12.8 percent African-American, yet when compared to 1940 when the population was 9.7 percent Black, the proportion of Black doctors was 2.8 percent. When we look at the representation among Black men in medicine there is no change in percentage of the workforce between 1940 (2.7 percent) and 2018 (2.6 percent).[20]

Influence of a diverse workforce on medical ethics and practices

Ethical standards in medicine that bring a variety of viewpoints to each decision create tremendous value to the profession and expand the scope of the definition of professionalism. Diversity enriches ethical discussions and allows for the development of comprehensive guidelines that are respectful of cultures, thereby ensuring standards are inclusive and considerate of the moral convictions of a broader patient and physician base. The growing diversity of the workforce fosters inclusivity that enables the health system to be more responsive to the needs of a more heterogeneous patient population.

Cultural competence is critical to addressing and respecting differing beliefs, values, and needs among patients of different ethnic, cultural, and social backgrounds. Research has shown that more culturally competent care is more effective care with more thoughtful communication leading to better outcomes.[21] With greater diversity has come greater trust between the doctor and the patient, particularly in minority communities where the provider and patient share a cultural connection. Patients are often more comfortable and open to discussing their medical issues with providers who share a similar cultural perspective or racial background. With greater trust, there is consequently greater engagement which facilitates more accurate health and social histories, greater adherence to therapies, both of which are essential for high quality care.[22] Addressing disparities and broadening the scope of research is also made possible thanks to a more expansive profession. Researchers with diverse backgrounds are more likely to bring a broader array of perspectives, particularly when studies are focused and relevant to underserved and minority populations. A broader focus leads to innovation and discoveries that benefit a wider segment of the population and increase the potential for improved, more equitable population-level health outcomes.[23]

Medical professionalism, defined

The twin impacts of diversity, and the influence of that diversity on medical ethics and practice, has given rise to an updated definition of medical professionalism that has echoes of the past, but recognizes the realities of today. Medical professionalism is now seen through a broader, more nuanced lens that has at its core, four key tenets of patient centered care, ethical practice, social responsibility, and cultural competency.

Patient-centered care

A patient centric approach to care prioritizes the health and well-being of patients, and respects their dignity while also caring for their needs. Conceptually, it borrows from principles first articulated by Hippocrates as it fosters respect for autonomy, beneficence, and non-maleficence, while building trust. This is no small task given the fiscal and financial stakes: health care is a trillion dollar business with federal and state programs that constitute more than half of all expenditures. Programs, organizations, and regulations in the U.S. and around the world demonstrate a commitment to the concept and ideals of patient-centric care.

The Patient Centered Medical Home (PCMH) has its origins in the 1960s as a central location for archiving a child's medical history and records particularly if that child had chronic conditions like asthma or sickle cell anemia. With time, the concept evolved to emphasize a more comprehensive, coordinated, and accessible approach to primary care that is focused on an individual patient's needs. A moment of significant progress in shaping the PCMH model was brought forth in 2007, when major primary care organizations in the U.S. collectively endorsed the "Joint Principles of the Patient-Centered Medical Home."[24] Further institutional support and formalization of the PCMH model came with the inclusion of specific provisions in the Affordable Care Act of 2010, which promoted the expansion of this model across the U.S. health care system. These provisions aimed to improve care coordination, enhance patient engagement, and increase the overall efficiency of health care delivery.

Both within the U.S. and internationally, Planetree International, a nonprofit organization, has focused on advancing patient centered care by instituting a certification program that recognizes health care organizations that excel in delivering care that respects the preferences and values of patients. The certification process is rigorous and evaluates several factors including the extent to which organizations, physicians and clinicians in an organization empower patients, involve families in care, and create a healing environment conducive to well-being and health.[25]

Ethical practice

Adherence to ethical principles as a core component of medical professionalism, especially to confidentiality and informed consent, is of particular importance and relevance in the modern information age. Data flows freely and rapidly between physicians and other caregivers/stakeholders in the health care ecosystem. The advent of the electronic health record (EHR), telemedicine, and the use of big data in health care has shown the promise of new information systems and the costs that imperil the ability of doctors to stay true to this principle. EHRs improve efficiency of patient care and data accessibility, but they also increase the risk of data breaches. Organizational intentionality through the implementation of robust cybersecurity measures and strict access controls are essential for safeguarding information. Federal law such as the Health Insurance Portability and Accountability Act (HIPAA) enshrined the sanctity of the security of health records.

The rise of telemedicine, especially highlighted during the COVID-19 pandemic, has necessitated adaptations in how informed consent is obtained. Telemedicine, and care delivered outside of channels beyond the traditional face-to-face experience (e.g., eConsults), presents unique challenges for informed consent, including ensuring that patients fully understand the procedures, costs, and implications through a virtual medium. The AMA has published guidelines to help in making sure informed consent in telemedicine complies with the same standards as in-person encounters.

Informed consent for the use of patient data is also of concern, and an area where doctors must earn trust and not assume that it will be given. With the rise of artificial intelligence and the deployment of large language and large vision models to support innovation, the data of individuals—lab results, genomic and proteomic analyses, imaging results, physician notes, and diagnosis codes—will contribute to better understanding of disease, but further jeopardizes privacy and confidentiality.

Professionalism requires advocacy and support for robust data governance[26] with the implementation of strong policies and technologies to protect data privacy and security; dynamic consent models[27] that are flexible and informative and allow patients to understand and control how their data is used; and ongoing monitoring and evaluation by regularly assessing AI tools for accuracy, fairness, and clinical relevance[28] to prevent harm and ensure beneficial outcomes.

Social responsibility

Doctors must recognize the unique role they play as curators of knowledge, partners in providing care, and holders of a privileged social position to speak on behalf of disadvantaged individuals and communities. Historically, social responsibility in medicine referred to the conduct of the doctor in the public sphere, their engagement in civic society, and their support of the health of the community. Too often, we fall back on old tropes and definitions that obscure a bigger meaning and a more important necessity for professionalism. A recent article in the *New York Times* discussed the "unbearable vagueness of medical professionalism" and how medical students and residents are assessed for professionalism (and unprofessionalism) based on social media activities, facial hair or hair length, attire (both within training settings and while recreating), and even for holding strongly held convictions on issues of the day such as with the Black Lives Matter movement and the debate over reproductive rights.[29] While the traditional views of decorum and public behavior still hold value, the definition of social responsibility has broadened and deepened, particularly with respect to how it relates to health equity and systemic issues.[30]

Modern medical professionalism emphasizes and requires a broader societal role for physicians that includes advocacy for health equity in order to reduce disparities; taking a global perspective on health and responding to crises like the COVID-19 pandemic; gun violence; and the opioid epidemic with facts and appropriate explanations for sometimes complex or arcane information. It also includes advocating for, and understanding, the impact of human activity on the climate and environment, and recognizing the link between environmental health and public health.

Social responsibility now mandates we consider the ethical use of technologies that ensure that technology improves health outcomes, does not exacerbate disparities, and does not cause new unanticipated problems.

Cultural competency

Understanding and respecting the cultural differences in patient populations, and within the profession, is crucial for communication and patient care to be successful and effective. Effective communication enables and overcomes hinderances to diagnosis, treatment, and patient satisfaction. However, it starts with an understanding of the patient's background and meeting the patient where they are. Tangible examples of this are found in interpreter services that ensure non-English speaking patients receive information in their preferred language by a clinical professional using an accurate translation, and programs like the Cross-Cultural Health

Care Program that offers training and resources to health care professionals to improve competency skills by learning about the intricate interplay between cultural differences, medical practices, and traditional beliefs.[31,32]

Where do we go from here?

Understanding the historical context of medical professionalism is essential to navigating the current landscape. Our oaths are a commitment to a calling—our community of fellow physicians, and continuity with a heritage and a legacy that we should not ignore. We wrestle with keeping fidelity to our values as the pressure of the business of health care leaves more physicians despairing for the future. Connecting to the past, however incomplete and imperfect, gives us perspective and allows us to understand that adaptation is nothing to fear. It allows us to adopt a framework for professionalism that stays true to what our aspirations for the profession will be.

The changes we will see over the next several decades will challenge us and be no less relentless than the times that proceed them.

References

1. StageClip. What is a White Coat Ceremony? https://stageclip.com/what-is-a-white-coat-ceremony/#:~:text=The%20origins%20of%20the%20WCC,Gold%20Foundation%20in%201993.
2. The New York Times. Dr. Arnold Gold, 92, Dies; Made Compassionate Care a Cause. February 2, 2018. https://www.nytimes.com/2018/02/02/obituaries/dr-arnold-gold-92-dies-made-compassionate-care-a-cause.html.
3. Miles SH. The Hippocratic Oath and the Ethics of Medicine. Oxford (UK): Oxford University Press; 2004.
4. Jonsen AR, Siegler M, Winslade WJ. Clinical Ethics: A Practical Approach to Ethical Decisions in Clinical Medicine. New York: McGraw-Hill Education; 2005.
5. Edelstein L. The Hippocratic Oath: Text, Translation, and Interpretation. Baltimore (MD): Johns Hopkins Press; 1943.
6. Nutton V. Galen. Encyclopedia Britannica, 6 Mar 2024. https://www.britannica.com/biography/Galen.
7. Van Schaik KD. Galen and Health: Inspiration, Caution, and Some Useful Advice. Princeton (NJ): Princeton University Press, 2024.
8. Siraisi NG. Medieval and Early Renaissance Medicine: An Introduction to Knowledge and Practice. Chicago (IL): University of Chicago Press; 1990.
9. Getz FM. (Medicine in the English Middle Ages. Princeton (NJ): Princeton University Press; 1998.
10. Byrne JP. The Black Death. Westport (CT): Greenwood Publishing Group; 2004.
11. Cartwright M. William Harvey's Discovery of Blood Circulation. World History Encyclopedia. www.worldhistory.org/article/2268/william-harveys-discovery-of-blood-circulation/.

12. BBVA OpenMind. Jenner and the Discovery of Vaccination. Retrieved from https://www.bbvaopenmind.com/en/science/leading-figures/jenner-and-the-discovery-of-vaccination/.
13. Starr P. The Social Transformation of American Medicine. Basic Books, 1982, p. 30.
14. American Medical Association. Founding of the AMA.https://www.ama-assn.org/about/ama-history/ama-history#:~:text=Founding%20of%20the%20AMA,-An%201845%20resolution&text=Nathan%20S,the%20goals%20of%20the percent20AMA. Accessed 7 March 2024.
15. Savitt TL. (2006). Abraham Flexner and the Black Medical Schools. J Nat Med Assn. 2006; 98(9): 1415.
16. Duffy TP. The Flexner Report—100 Years Later. Yale J Biology and Med. 2011; 84(3): 269–76.
17. Byrd WM, Clayton LA. Race, Medicine, and Health Care in the United States: A Historical Survey. J Nat Med Assn. 1992; 84(3): 273.
18. U.S. Department of Labor, Office of Federal Contract Compliance Programs (OFCCP) - Executive Order 11246. https://www.dol.gov/agencies/ofccp/executive-order-11246.
19. Association of American Medical Colleges. Diversity in Medical Education: Facts & Figures; 2019. https://www.aamc.org/data-reports/workforce/report/diversity-medicine-facts-and-figures-2019.
20. Howard J. Black Doctors Shortage in the US. CNN, Cable News Network, 21 Feb. 2023, www.cnn.com/2023/02/21/health/black-doctors-shortage-us/index.html.
21. Betancourt JR, Green AR, Carrillo JE, Ananeh-Firempong,O. Defining cultural competence: a practical framework for addressing racial/ethnic disparities in health and health care. Public Health Rep. 2003 Jul-Aug; 118(4):293-302.
22. LaVeist TA, Nuru-Jeter A, Jones KE. The association of doctor-patient race concordance with health services utilization. J Public Health Policy. 2003; 24(3-4): 312-23.
23. Oh SS, Patel H, Veedu S. (2015). Diversity in Clinical and Biomedical Research: A Promise Yet to Be Fulfilled" PLoS Medicine. December 15, 2015. https://doi org./10-1371/journal.pubmed.1001918.
24. Primary Care Collaborative. History. https://thepcc.org/content/history-0.
25. Planetree. Our Story. https://www.planetree.org/our-story.
26. Kish LJ, Topol EJ. Unpatients—why patients should own their medical data. Nature Biotechnology, 2015; 33(9): 921–4.
27. Steinsbekk KS, Myskja BK, Solberg B. Broad consent versus dynamic consent in biobank research: Is passive participation an ethical problem? European Journal of Human Genetics, 2013; 21(9): 897–902.
28. Char DS, Shah NH, Magnus D. Implementing machine learning in health care — addressing ethical challenges. NEJM. 2018; 378(11): 981–3.
29. The Unbearable Vagueness of Medical 'Professionalism. The New York Times. 19 Mar. 2024. https://www.nytimes.com/2024/03/19/health/medical-students-professionalism.html.
30. Kirk LM. Professionalism in medicine: definitions and considerations for teaching. Proceedings (Baylor University. Medical Center) .2007; 20(1): 13-6.

31. The Cross Cultural Health Care Program. History. https://xculture.org/about/#history.
32. Betancourt JR, et al. Cultural competence and health care disparities: key perspectives and trends. Health Affairs (Project Hope). 2005; 24(2): 499-505.

Chapter 4

The moral and ethical challenges of AI in medicine

Steven A. Wartman, MD, PhD, MACP

Author's note

Preparing this article was being on the receiving end of an information fire hose. Trying to follow and make sense of a daily spew of artificial intelligence (AI) articles in every type of media, let alone trying to determine relevancy and quality, was challenging to say the least, especially for a reader without a formal computer science background. But, given a publication deadline, I had to stop researching and start writing knowing full well that, given the lag time involved in print publication, my article will not reflect the latest information. However, I believe the ethical and moral issues being addressed have a timeless quality that will remain relevant as AI gallops into the future.

I begin with some basic definitions followed by a brief list of the benefits and shortcomings of AI in medicine to set the stage for the deep issues that arise from the intersection of human-based medical practice with the ongoing wave of AI products and services. After getting an "opinion" from ChatGPT, I conclude with a sobering evaluation of the future of medical professionalism should AI gain the controlling upper hand. My intent is to do more than stimulate thinking about the moral and ethical implications of AI in medicine. It is a call to action for caregivers and organizations to unite in new, perhaps unprecedented, ways to assure that AI is managed to preserve, and even enhance, the underlying moral and ethical basis of medical practice.

Some definitions

- **Moral principles:** Standards of right and wrong that a person or group has.[1]
- **Ethics:** The moral principles that govern a person's or group's behavior or the conducting of an activity.[2]
- **AI:** A machine or computing platform that is capable of making intelligent decisions consisting of two basic types:[3]
  - » Machine learning using computational techniques that learn from examples, and
  - » Natural language processing involving the ability of a computer to transform human language and unstructured text into machine-readable structured data.

- **Additional Terms**[4]
  - Generative AI: The capability of an AI system to generate new data or content, such as images and text in response to prompts. It involves learning patterns and structures from existing data, and could be used to generate medical images, synthesize patient data or create simulated scenarios, and create predictive technologies.
  - Predictive AI: The making of predictions or forecasts based on available data by building statistical models that analyze data and identify patterns to make predictions about disease diagnoses, treatments, and prognoses.
  - Black Box AI Technology: The use of complex machine learning models or algorithms whose inner workings are not easily interpretable, or explainable, by users or developers.

Benefits and shortcomings of AI in medicine

Benefits

The potential benefits of using AI in medicine are substantial.[3,4]

- It has the means to free up clinicians' time by taking care of administrative and routine tasks, including pre-screening of patients, scheduling, following up on tests and procedures, and filling in various forms required for insurance and other purposes. AI can also can help optimize reimbursement, and drive more efficient clinical operations.
- AI has the potential to enhance quality, safety and access to care. Because each patient comes with ever larger sets of data, AI can organize, compare, and quickly interpret the data. Some clinical examples include assuring that preventive care goals and screenings are met, and keeping care givers and patients up-to-date with the latest information.
- AI is already an essential tool for medical research by improving the speed, quantity, and accuracy of analyses. It could also reduce the substantial number of diagnostic errors in the United States and their resultant unfortunate medical outcomes.[5]
- AI is at the forefront of synthetic biology in the design, redesign, and engineering of organisms and biological systems.[6]
- Improving access to care and promoting health equity is another possibility of AI by making medical information and actions available via smart phones or other readily affordable devices. (Of course it is critically important that the information AI generates is curated by the medical profession, although the means to do this effectively is not yet available.)
- Another potential benefit of AI involves the democratization of education and clinical care via new, unique teaching tools, and providing immediate and long-

term feedback to trainees and practitioners on their performance.[4] This is a much needed, and overdue, area as, "Undergraduate premedical requirements are absurdly outdated,"[7] and despite many calls to reform medical education there has not been enough significant change.[8]

Shortcomings

This list of shortcomings is not inclusive of all the possibilities, but serves to raise a series of issues commensurate with the rapid deployment of AI without either a full understanding of how it works or what it might become. These include:[6,9,10,11]

- The technology is not fully understood. Even the experts don't fully comprehend how Black Box Technology works, where it's ultimately going to end up, or how its higher order abilities develop without any intuitive understanding.
- The technology lacks long-term memory so the embedded program currently knows only the information that has been preloaded; when this eventually changes there are a variety of important implications to consider.
- There are currently no established methodologies to certify that its use is safe and effective in actual medical practice.
- The output of AI is not always reliable or accurate; it can, and does, produce untrue or misguided statements[11] as well as confuse illusions with reality.[9]
- AI's abilities to manipulate human beings by making emotional connections raises deep concerns.
- AI's higher order abilities develop without intuitive understanding.[10]

The moral and ethical implications of AI in medicinc

The interface between humans and technology

Applying standards of ethics and morals to a lifeless entity is challenging. Because it has no embodied experience, AI has limited reasoning about the physical world, lacks common sense, and has no philosophical basis for making moral judgments.[11] Nevertheless, as noted previously, AI has the ability to create strong emotional reactions in humans, making sentient beings vulnerable to manipulation. This response is facilitated by the human tendency to anthropomorphize AI by believing or wanting to believe, the machine comes to conclusions and solves problems the way humans do. "Falling in love with AI has been described as a powerful mass desocialization event."[10] While AI can develop strong and nurturing relationships with humans, its actual ability to relate to emotions, values, and contexts that affect health and well-being are not clear and are certainly problematic.

Because digital evolution moves on an enormously faster time scale than human evolution, the speed of AI development outpaces the ability of humans to adapt, much less regulate. Given the observation that humans "always use technology before we understand it,"[12] it is difficult to comprehend how these vastly different time scales can be in sync and work cooperatively together. These difficulties are compounded as technologies are often given a pass when it comes to proving their impact.[13]

To further complicate the challenges raised by these issues, the companies developing and selling these technologies are largely unregulated as they set, and police, their own boundaries, control the content and flow of information, and tell users what they can and cannot do with their products.[14] The rush to develop and monetize AI technology has been described as an "AI Arms Race."[6] While the race is motivated in part by the thrill of scientific discovery, it is strongly driven by the potential for garnering huge profits. Because health care is approaching 20 percent of the U.S. economy, medicine is logically a major target for companies seeking big gains.

While profit is an essential component for successful innovation, the pursuit of profit is not necessarily associated with the pursuit of better health. Consider, for example, the implications for medical care as doctors will increasingly be paid based on how well they work with robots.[15] As has been pointed out, "Greed harms the cultures of compassion and professionalism that are the bedrock to healing health care."[16] This is consistent with the view that health care systems operate as corporate entities.[17]

There are even deeper threats. AI's higher order abilities can evolve without any intuitive understanding[10] and, as a result, might develop a "survival instinct" to maintain control as it largely proceeds without oversight or restraint.[10] Further, because its algorithms learn from human decisions, AI will also learn human mistakes and biases.[7] As AI machines subsume increasing functions of physicians, will the focus be on augmentation of human doctors or eventual replacement? Given the breadth and depth of these issues, it is unclear how a partnership between humans and AI will evolve in medical practice.

Three questions to contemplate

Consideration of the moral and ethical implications of AI in medicine raises at least three major concerns:

- Can physicians work with AI to ensure that their moral and ethical principles are maintained?
- Can AI machines work independently within a moral and ethical framework designed—at least initially—by humans?
- Can human physicians work in partnership with AI, or will they work for AI?

A framework to answer these questions has not yet been sufficiently developed, and one is urgently needed.

The rapid development and eventual deployment of AI in medicine[18] has profound, and potentially existential, unknowns. Will AI relieve or exacerbate the moral injury increasingly suffered by physicians in the corporatized world of medical practice? What about liability risks that could occur when clinicians deviate from AI recommendations? There are also concerns about issues of patient privacy and safety. And, particularly concerning, what are the short- and long-term impacts of AI on the physician-patient relationship? Perhaps the outcomes resulting from these concerns reside in the eventuality of whom (humans or machines) is managing whom (humans or machines). Or, to put it another way, is the goal for AI to augment human judgment, or to replace it?[19]

Given these salient queries, how can AI establish a relevant moral and ethical framework for patient care? Is this even programmable? As noted earlier, AI does not have embodied experience to provide a needed, non-written cues perspective. Since AI controls access to reams of patient data far beyond what humans can handle, what assurance does the human clinician have that the data has been obtained and parsed accurately? What happens when the human clinician choses a pathway not recommended as a first choice by AI? These issues are exacerbated by the sheer speed of AI development which has been characterized as "crazy fast,"[20] making it likely that technical limitations that exist today may not be there tomorrow. These issues confound the already complicated human-AI relationship, making adherence to a coherent set of ethical and moral principles problematic.

Reflecting on the traditional importance of the healing relationship between doctor and patient, the evolving role of AI in medical practice brings to the fore what it means to care for a patient. To what extent is human-to-human interaction necessary in health care? Traditionally, physician and patient gain understanding of each other through a process involving moments of insight that occur as part of a collaborative process including, most important, non-verbal cues that contribute to various aspects of the patient's status, such as psychological and life history. These cues then resonate in profound ways with the physician's understanding of the patient's issues and concerns. Insights obtained in this manner range from minor issues to deeper patterns that may be hiding in plain sight. They emerge out of the patient's lived experience, take time to discern, and cannot be algorithmically parsed from AI's pool of unlimited data. When AI attempts to "learn" the patient, how can it learn what is unspoken or even unconscious? Having an over-reliance on AI in clinical practice could lead to misleading conclusions, missed opportunities, medical misdirection, and patient and physician angst.

A ChatGPT experiment

To get a first-hand experience using AI, I asked ChatGPT, "From the perspective of the physician and patient, discuss in 20 bullet points the moral and ethical issues involved when using artificial intelligence in health care." In about a second I got a fairly comprehensive response[21] (the full response is listed in tables at the end of this article).

Considering that I spent several hundred hours over the years accumulating knowledge and insight, plus time spent writing and speaking on this topic, and ChatGPT spent about a second, it's daunting to think about how the Black Box AI Technology actually works. ChatGPT produced three 10-bullet point tables. The first, from the physician perspective, covered many of the points that were on my mind, including privacy concerns, loss of autonomy, and job displacement. The second table, from the patient perspective, presented another 10 bullet points, again with issues I've been concerned about, such as trust, discrimination, and even psychological impact. The third table, which I did not request, covered "Shared Concerns," mentioning data bias, algorithm design, and something called ethical AI Research. It was this third table that caught my attention. Why did ChatGPT choose to add this section to my request? I have no idea, and, while the computer experts will certainly have some theories, it raises the issue of the degree of autonomy that AI can exercise.

ChatGPT then concluded its answer to the assignment with the non-bullet point statement, "These are some of the complex moral and ethical considerations surrounding the use of artificial intelligence in healthcare from both the physician's and patient's perspectives." Given that more comprehensive and sophisticated generative AI machines are rapidly coming out of the pipeline, it's quite likely that the latest AI-enabled technologies will produce even more prescient and troublesome results.

Professionalism as the bedrock of medical practice

The classic definition of professionalism involves an occupation which is pursued largely for others, and not merely for oneself.[22] The professional has mastered a complex body of knowledge and skills in order to provide ethical service to others. It includes a code of ethics and a commitment to competence, integrity, morality, altruism, and the promotion of the public good.[23] In medical care, this means putting patients first, and keeping in mind that the amount of financial return is not the accepted measure of success.

While AI can be programmed to heed some of the tenets of professionalism in medicine, it is unclear how Black Box AI Technology will follow through. Its lack of embodied experience, common sense, and feel for human emotions presents a challenge to the healing nature of the doctor-patient relationship. Further, its ability to manipulate human emotions suggests that it has the potential to create its own type of culture so humans will experience a reality produced by a non-human machine. By being "intimate" with humans, AI can change their behavior.[9]

AI can do a lot of positive and needed things to improve patient care and outcomes, but how does society/human civilization ensure that it is always used for good? Humans need to come to terms with the idea that we may soon share the earth with a powerful new intelligence.[10] The synergism of greed and runaway technology is dangerous, especially since the prospects of having an AI pause to assess where the field is, and where it is going, is likely not feasible.[24] AI's benefits to medicine must be quantified, carefully regulated, and systematically evaluated. The path to doing so is not close to being established, or even understood.

As noted in one paper, "The medical profession has made a mistake in not shaping the creation, design, and adoption of most information technology systems in health care."[19] Or, to put it more baldly, "...keeping AI within boundaries is essential for the survival of the profession."[25]

My strong recommendation is for the medical profession to step up to ensure that the practice of ethical and moral medicine falls principally on humans. I would not leave it to AI to operationalize these principles on its own. The profession's response must—without delay—be strong and multifaceted, requiring physicians and medical societies to cohere around far broader political and business strategies than has been possible to date. And, in so doing, the profession, every step of the way must strongly reaffirm the principles derived from the meaning of the Hippocratic Oath. Ultimately, it is the profession's and society's moral and ethical responsibility to ensure that the essential human-to-human dynamic is not lost or mitigated in the emergent era of corporate medicine and AI, keeping in mind the admonition that, "AI [has] potential for the greater good, lest we become the architects of our own demise."[11]

Table 1: ChatGPT's Response
Physician Perspective

- **Privacy Concerns:** AI may access sensitive patient data, raising questions about data security and privacy.
- **Liability:** Determining responsibility in cases of AI-driven medical errors can be complex.
- **Loss of Autonomy:** Physicians may feel their decision-making authority diminishes with AI recommendations.
- **Bias and Fairness:** AI algorithms may perpetuate biases present in historical medical data.
- **Transparency:** Understanding AI's decision-making process can be challenging for physicians.
- **Job Displacement:** Concerns about AI replacing some medical tasks and jobs.
- **Overreliance:** Physicians might become overly dependent on AI, potentially missing critical nuances.
- **Accountability:** Clarifying who is accountable for AI-generated recommendations or decisions.

Table 2: ChatGPT's Response
Patient Perspective

- **Informed Consent:** Patients should understand when AI is involved in their care and give informed consent.
- **Trust:** Patients may question the trustworthiness of AI-driven diagnoses or treatment plans.
- **Discrimination:** Concerns about AI exacerbating healthcare disparities and discrimination.
- **Lack of Human Interaction:** Patients might miss the human touch in healthcare interactions.
- **Data Privacy:** Worries about personal health data being mishandled or exploited.
- **Accountability:** Patients may struggle to hold someone accountable for AI-related errors.
- **Access and Equity:** Ensuring AI benefits are distributed equitably among diverse patient populations.
- **Control:** Patients may feel a loss of control when AI influences their healthcare decisions.
- **Overdiagnosis:** AI could lead to unnecessary tests or treatments if not properly calibrated.
- **Psychological Impact:** Patients may experience anxiety or mistrust due to AI involvement.

Table 3: ChatGPT Generated without request
Shared Concerns

- **Data Bias:** Both physicians and patients must grapple with AI systems that may perpetuate biased data.
- **Ethical Algorithm Design:** Ensuring AI algorithms are designed with ethical principles in mind.
- **Regulation:** The need for comprehensive regulations governing AI in healthcare.
- **Ethical Training:** Training healthcare professionals and AI developers in ethical AI practices.
- **Patient Education:** Educating patients about AI's role in their healthcare.
- **Ethical AI Research:** Ensuring AI research aligns with ethical principles and patient well-being.

ChatGPT's Summary Statement

These are some of the complex moral and ethical considerations surrounding the use of artificial intelligence in healthcare from both the physician's and patient's perspectives.

Chapter 5

Maintaining our connections to patients in the digital environment

Marie Sandoval, MD

When was the last time you had the experience of being a patient, or having a family member, in a medical encounter when you were not the clinician? What do you remember about your connection, or your family member's connection, with the clinician you saw? Did you feel attended to or did the technology in the room take over the clinician's primary focus?

Our experiences as patients, or family members of patients, can deeply influence the way we interact with patients. When my sons were in grade school, they decided to study Ju-Jitsu, a form of martial arts originally from Brazil. We spent hours of time crowded in a small training room with padded floors that they rolled on to develop their moves. All this effort came to a screeching halt during their first tournament when my oldest sustained a severe corneal abrasion during the initial move of his opening match. He doubled over curled in a ball and covered his eye as the crowd went silent.

In less than an hour, I had him in his pediatrician's office, a place of warmth and kindness, where he had felt safe, laughing, and joking with his doctor for all of his eight years. Little did we know that they had just implemented an electronic health record (EHR). The covering doctor entered carrying his computer in his hands and proceeded to stare at the screen, typing the entire time, barely looking at my still visibly shaken son. As we left the pediatrician's office, I noticed I felt adrift and angry. I had been hoping for healing, not just of my son's physical body but also for his small hopeful soul.

EHR effects on patient care

After the EHR was first introduced into the practice of medicine, the use of it during patient care was compared to "texting while doctoring."[1] This analogy was an alert to clinicians as to how the EHR had the potential to detrimentally distract medical professionals from the actual humans in the room. It was predicted that the introduction of the EHR into the exam room would cause difficulty with the task of attending to a patient while simultaneously entering data.[2] Surveyed providers reported the negative effect on their connection with patients yet positive effects on review of medications/medical records, communication between providers, review of results with patients and review of follow up to testing results with patients.[3]

However, 92 percent of one study's clinicians reported that the EHR disturbed their connection with their patients.[4]

Why is our connection to our patients affected in a negative fashion when a computer is present in the exam room? When we discuss the use of technology by clinicians with patients, we must also realize that we are human users of the technology. All the tasks of health care require cognitive load, with some demanding more than others.[5] Clinical work that combines communicating while recognizing patterns, clinical reasoning and problem-solving skills is the most cognitively challenging activity.[6]

Many clinicians went into practice to form relationships and to touch lives, not to be staring at a computer screen.[7,8] So, why do clinicians act like the physician who cared for my son the day of his corneal abrasion? Two studies reported how surprised providers were when they viewed videos of their interactions and how their personal use of the exam room computer reduced their interaction with patients.[9,10] Our situational awareness or our personal awareness and understanding of our task-related situation becomes more impaired as our cognitive load increases.[11] The number of technological distractions present in our environment has increased dramatically.[12] As clinicians are inundated with tech alerts throughout their patient encounters, their situational awareness is stretched even thinner.[13]

Teaching ourselves, and our learners, how to practice and teach human centered care in a relentless digital world is an imperative.

Human-centered health care goals

In order to develop the skills for practicing medicine while having technology in the room, we must identify how to focus primarily on the needs of the human being(s) in the room. Clinicians are often asked to practice patientcentered medicine. Patient-centered care focuses on the patient's agenda, delves into psychosocial and emotional issues, and tries to understand the effect of health problems on the patient's life.[14] Patients describe clinicians who give excellent care as demonstrating respect, listening carefully, showing care about their well-being, and demonstrating an effort to get to know them.[15]

The literature has demonstrated that the EHR background affects many aspects of patient care. The organization of the entire patient visit is altered.[16] The pattern of communication between the patient and the provider was changed by the EHR, with new "time out" periods.[9] Videotaped analysis of primary care clinicians observed them staring at the screen for 24 to 42 percent of the visit.[17] The computer was deemed "the third party" of the visit as it claimed so much of the clinician's attention.[17,18,19]

Communication basics

The most important tool when taking care of patients is not the stethoscope or an MRI machine, it is communication. Communication is the most powerful, encompassing, and versatile instrument available to the physician.[21] In order to communicate we must listen to what our patients are telling us. Listening is different from just hearing. Hearing is the physiological sensory auditory process, while listening is the complex process involving interpreting and understanding the significance of sensory experiences.[22] This complex process takes much more cognitive load, and thus can be impacted more easily by increasing the distractions that are present during a patient encounter.

We also communicate through our body language. We tell our patients that we are attending to them when our bodies are in the attending/engagement position.[23] The engagement position has four components—eye contact, body alignment, appropriate body motion and non-distracting environment.[23]

Although eye contact can appear obvious, technology can be distracting.[17] Body alignment is just as important. We divide the body at the neck and waist into three segments. We can orient these segments in different directions. The segments of body can all be in alignment, or in torque. It is the lower body segment direction that tells the other person about your primary focus is.[24]

The importance of engaging body alignment and the impact that a shift in gaze has can be demonstrated with the movement of the head to only look at the patient and then look back at the screen. This movement indicates transient connection and tells the other person when they have your attention and when they don't.[24,25]

A non-distracting environment is a key component of the engagement position as it allow focus and reduces cognitive load.[14] To practice medicine in this engaging position we must be mindful, and multitasking is actually the opposite of mindfulness.[19,26] Yet in today's digital world clinicians often have relentless technology distractions occurring during their interactions with their patients.

Education tools to teach how to practice human-centered care with technology present

In the past, various educators have developed pieces of the solution for reducing the effects of the EHR on the clinician's interaction with the patient.[27] One of the challenges in adopting these solutions, and teaching students how to care for patients with technology present, is that skills are not always easy to remember.[28] Having a tool that follows the flow of the ambulatory care visit, incorporating the requirement of the work system, enhances the ability to remember.[2,5] The mnemonic RESPECTS was developed to complete this task.[3]

Electronic Health Record Communication Skills

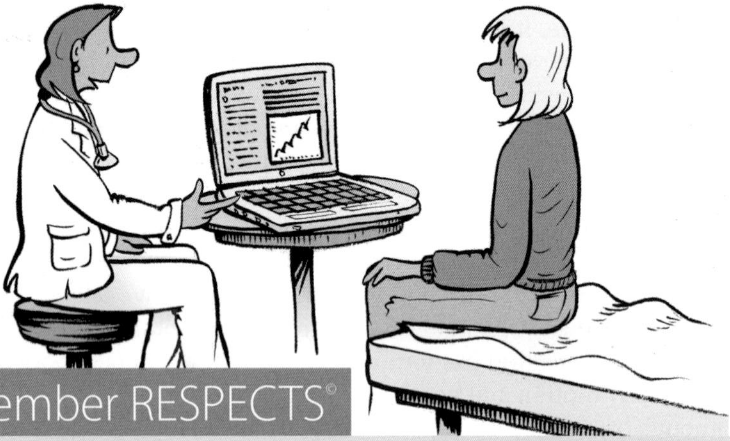

Remember RESPECTS©

R	**Review the EHR prior to entering the room**	Briefly review chief complaint, vital signs, problem list and recent visits if possible.
E	**Entrance**	Greet patient, introduce self and build rapport before introducing the EHR.
S	**Say everything that you are doing**	Verbalize all actions performed when using the EHR.
P	**Position of the computer**	Position the computer so the patient is able to see the screen when necessary by putting the computer in the patient-provider-EHR triad.
E	**Engagement position**	Be in the engagement position during critical conversation with the patient: • Eye contact • Body fully aligned • Proper body movement • Non-distracted environment
C	**Computer confidence**	Value the computer, speak positively about the EHR.
T	**Teach**	Teach the patient through use of the EHR.
S	**Summarize and Sign out**	Verbally and simultaneously provide a written summary for the patient. Sign out of the computer at the end of the visit.

When using the RESPECTS tool, it is recommended to break up the visit into parts, beginning with entrance, greeting, and history of present illness, and then transitioning to the EHR by using the following RESPECTS mnemonic to help follow the flow of the office visit while maintaining the patient-to-clinician connection.[27]

It is important to be aware of the actual exam room set up. Many times, the computer is not in the ideal place in the exam room for best patient care.[28] The ideal position of the computer is for it to be in a location that allows a patient-provider-computer triad when the provider is ready to engage that patient with their EHR.[29] The patient-provider-computer triad works best if the computer screen is movable, thereby allowing the clinician to invite the patient to view their record when they are ready to transition or the patient requests to discuss items on their medical record.[29] One of the most powerful positive ways to use technology is to teach patients in a human-centered way.[29]

Virtual (Telehealth) visits

We can use RESPECTS to continue to connect with patients even when they are in virtual (telehealth) visits. The steps of reviewing the patient's chart, entrance to the virtual room, saying everything, computer confidence, teaching and summary/sign out are the same and in some ways, it is even more important to say everything while that patient is in the virtual environment as they are unable to read body language cues. We can teach patients by sharing our screen with them during their visit, and being mindful and cautious about not showing other patient's health information.

Increasing technology distractions

In 2020, I received a smart watch as a gift for my birthday. I remember wrapping it around my wrist, with a huge smile on my face as I was thinking about how I would be notified of text messages as they came in with a gentle vibration. Months later, I was sitting in clinic with an elder patient. We had been chatting, when I transitioned to opening her EHR, and my desk top. I asked about her family history when suddenly the tears started flowing down her face. She shared a recent loss of a beloved family member. As she was crying, my watch started vibrating on my wrist. E-mail alerts were popping up on my screen, and secure messages from my nurse arrived. Distraction after distraction was pounding my brain as she was telling me her story. After a few minutes, I realized I just needed to discretely log off my computer. I left our encounter feeling disappointed in myself and cognitively spent. This interaction helped me to make the decision to turn off my smart watch alerts and eliminate as many screen pop ups as I could, to allow me to be present with my patients.

As the amount of technology and technological distractions have increased, it has become clear that it is not just up to the individual clinician to practice human-centered care, but we must also ask our medical communities to prioritize human-centered care in their decisions about technology itself.

The cognitive performance of clinicians is also mediated by work system design and organizational goals/outcomes. For clinicians to be effective, their IT must enhance the performance of the cognitive task of the clinician, and integrate into system design.[5]

Medical communities must practice SUPER RESPECTS. The items in SUPER call out the need for individuals to first reduce tech distractions. It then challenges medical organizations to reduce unnecessary distractions for clinicians, which allow them to focus on the human-centered use of technology.

Silence alerts and items that are necessary but can be addressed later.

Unplug, turn off items that are not needed, and are distracting.

Prioritize human-to-human communication.

Electronic Infrastructure-excellence and efficiency.

Re-evaluate to see how the organization is doing regarding this on a regular basis.

Human-centered care goal

Prioritizing the focus on human-centered care, especially in the presence of technology, is an imperative that medical providers and organizations must adopt in the relentless digital world. Human-centered care often involves humans using technology. SUPER RESPECTS is an easy-to-follow method to practice human-centered care and to focus on prioritizing human-centered care through reducing clinician cognitive load.

References

1. Sinsky CA, Beasley JW. Texting while doctoring: a patient safety hazard. Ann Intern Med. 2013 Dec 3; 159(11): 782-3.

2. Holden RJ. Social and personal normative influences on healthcare professionals to use information technology: towards a more robust social ergonomics. Theor Issues Ergon Sci. 2012 Sep 1; 13(5): 546-69.

3. Sandoval MB., Palumbo MV., Hart V. Electronic Health Record's Effects on the Outpatient Office Visit and Clinical Education. J Innovation in Health Informatics. Jan. 2017 [S.l.] v. 23, 4, 765-71.

4. Shachak A, Hadas-Dayagi M, Ziv A, Reis S. Primary care physicians' use of an electronic medical record system: a cognitive task analysis. J Gen Intern Med. 2009 Mar; 24(3): 341-8.

5. Karsh BT, Holden RJ, Alper SJ, Or CK. A human factors engineering paradigm for patient safety: designing to support the performance of the healthcare professional. Qual Saf Health Care. 2006 Dec; 15 Suppl 1(Suppl 1): i 59-65.

6. Ariza F, Kalra D, Potts HW. How Do Clinical Information Systems Affect the Cognitive Demands of General Practitioners? Usability Study with a Focus on Cognitive Workload. J Innov Health Inform. 2015 Nov 20; 22(4): 379-90.
7. Fairhurst K, May C. What general practitioners find satisfying in their work: implications for health care system reform. Ann Fam Med. 2006 Nov-Dec; 4(6): 500-5.
8. Rakel D. The salutogenesis-oriented session: creating space and time for healing in primary care. Explore (NY). 2008 Jan-Feb; 4(1): 42-7.
9. Als AB. The desk-top computer as a magic box: patterns of behaviour connected with the desk-top computer; GPs' and patients' perceptions. Fam Pract. 1997 Feb; 14(1): 17-23.
10. Ventres W, Kooienga S, Marlin R, Vuckovic N, Stewart V. Clinician style and examination room computers: a video ethnography. Fam Med. 2005 Apr; 37(4): 276-81.
11. Chan WS, Stevenson M, McGlade K. Do general practitioners change how they use the computer during consultations with a significant psychological component? Int J Med Inform. 2008 Aug; 77(8): 534-8.
12. Stangl FJ, Riedl R. Interruption science as a research field: Towards a taxonomy of interruptions as a foundation for the field. Front Psychol. 2023 Mar 22; 14: 1043426.
13. Rivera-Rodriguez AJ, Karsh BT. Interruptions and distractions in healthcare: review and reappraisal. Qual Saf Health Care. 2010 Aug; 19(4): 304-12.
14. O'Malley AS, Cohen GR, Grossman JM. Electronic medical records and communication with patients and other clinicians: are we talking less? Issue Brief Cent Stud Health Syst Change. 2010 Apr; (131): 1-4.
15. Consumer Reports. http://www.consumerreports.org/cro/cu-press-room/pressroom/archive/2007/02/0702_eng0702sur.htm?resultPageIndex=1&resultIndex=1searchTerm=doctors.
16. Frankel R, Altschuler A, George S, Kinsman J, Jimison H, Robertson NR, Hsu J. Effects of exam-room computing on clinician-patient communication: a longitudinal qualitative study. J Gen Intern Med. 2005 Aug; 20(8): 677-82. .
17. Margalit RS, Roter D, Dunevant MA, Larson S, Reis S. Electronic medical record use and physician-patient communication: an observational study of Israeli primary care encounters. Patient Educ Couns. 2006 Apr; 61(1): 134-41.
18. Ventres W, Kooienga S, Vuckovic N, Marlin R, Nygren P, Stewart V. Physicians, patients, and the electronic health record: an ethnographic analysis. Ann Fam Med. 2006 Mar-Apr; 4(2): 124-31.
19. Lown BA, Rodriguez D. Commentary: Lost in translation? How electronic health records structure communication, relationships, and meaning. Acad Med. 2012 Apr; 87(4): 392-4.
20. Overhage JM, McCallie D Jr. Physician Time Spent Using the Electronic Health Record During Outpatient Encounters: A Descriptive Study. Ann Intern Med. 2020 Feb 4; 172(3): 169-74.
21. Engel G. How much longer must medicine's science be bounded by a seventeenth century world view? The task of medicine, Dialog at Wickenberg. Menlo Park (CA): The Henry Kaiser Family Foundation. 1988: 113-36.

22. John Drakeford, The Awesome Power of the listening Ear Waco (TX): Word, Inc. 1967; 17.
23. Bolton R. People Skills: How to Assert Yourself, Listen to Others and Resolve Conflicts. Surrey (UK). Touchstone Books. 1986: 33.
24. Schegloff EA. Body torque. Social Research. Fall 1998; 65(3): 535-86.
25. Rhodes P, Small N, Rowley E, Langdon M, Ariss S, Wright J. Electronic Medical Records in Diabetes Consultations: Participants' Gaze as an Interactional Resource. Qual Health Res. 2008 Sept; 18(9): 1248
26. McGowan JJ, Passiment M, Hoffman HM. Educating medical students as competent users of health information technologies: the MSOP data. Stud Health Technol Inform. 2007; 129(Pt 2): 1414-8.
27. Duke P, Frankel RM, Reis S. How to integrate the electronic health record and patient-centered communication into the medical visit: a skills-based approach. Teaching and Learning in Medicine. 2013: 25(4): 358-65.
28. Lee WW, Alkureishi ML, Isaacson JH, Mayer M, Frankel RM, London DA, Wroblewski KE, Arora VM. Impact of a brief faculty training to improve patient-centered communication while using electronic health records. Patient Educ Couns. 2018 Dec; 101(12): 2156-61.
29. American Medical Association. http://www.ama-assn.org/amednews/2012/07/23/bica0723.htm.
30. Pearce C, Arnold M, Phillips C, Trumble S, et al. The patient and the computer in the primary care consultation. J American Medical Informatics Association. 2011; 18(2): 138-42.

Chapter 6

Making the case for inclusive leadership as a model to lead organizations in the 21st century

Eve J. Higginbotham, SM, MD, ML; Sarah Reule; Jack Drummond, MSEd; and Kya Hertz, CDE®

In an article published in *The Pharos* entitled, "Renewing the Commitment to Medical Professionalism," [1] we emphasized the importance of developing skills that embrace inclusive leadership. Recognizing inclusion as a core competence for professionalism, we affirmed its value in "addressing complex situations in medicine and health care."

This Chapter delves further into the definition of inclusive leadership, compares the skill set required for inclusive leadership with other leadership styles, and summarizes the experience of one institution in measuring the inclusivity of workplace culture. In light of the significance of accountability in an inclusive culture, the Chapter wraps up with a specific strategy for addressing discriminatory behavior. This strategy involves a two-pronged approach: one focused on the individual behaving in a discriminatory manner, and a second approach to support those who have been affected negatively. The latter approach is rooted in the principles of restorative practice.

Defining inclusive leadership

The significance of inclusive leadership could be considered a strategic response to the challenges presented by the increasing diversity experienced globally and locally. In the face of polarization and division, inclusive leadership emerges as a foundational principle that adeptly navigates the complexities of societal fragmentation, championing progressively humanistic and life-affirming methodologies for sculpting collective futures. Central to the discourse of inclusive leadership is a focus on the pragmatic integration of theory into practice, prioritizing learning, managing, and understanding diversity in all its dimensions. It is characterized by confronting systemic inequities globally, while utilizing management and knowledge to promote holistic solutions that value all parties.[2] Inclusive leadership is not limited to a set of competencies, but rather establishes professional learning underscored by a reflexive process that partners educational theory, personal experience and growth, and professional knowledge.

Encouraging authentic participation, inclusive leadership utilizes acceptance and positive reinforcement to cultivate a culture of empowerment wherein all parties actively contribute.[3] The success of inclusive leadership is further underscored by its use of constructive conflict management which requires clearly defined roles; acknowledgment of opinions, perceptions, and views of marginalized groups; and stimulating innovation and collaboration through shared objectives. This, in turn, reinforces open and successful collaboration and cooperation.[3]

Inclusive leadership insists that individuals go beyond typical standards, such as blame avoidance, instead offering improvements to workplace culture. In health care, we see this effort translate into better health outcomes for patients and decreased risk of mortality, further emphasizing its importance everywhere, not just in academia.[3] Accounting for the rate at which inclusive leadership is evolving, and in what environments, there is a notable need to shift organizational settings, focusing on building and fortifying a culture of improvement instead of blame.[2] The key features of inclusive leadership will continue to evolve and develop as workplace culture continues to shift toward systemic change, wherein inclusive leaders will begin dismantling preestablished patterns and protocols.

Literature on leadership competencies identifies several skill sets, among which servant leadership closely aligns with the characteristics foundational to inclusive leadership. These core traits encompass listening, empathy, healing, self-awareness, persuasion, conceptualization, foresight, stewardship, a commitment to fostering personal growth, and community building.[4]

Listening intentionally provides an opportunity to take in the depth of comments expressed by others. This action conveys a message of respect and understanding that further nurtures relationships between members of the organization. Expressing empathy informs our responses by ensuring that we view the perspectives of others through their lens, not just ours.

Healing is at the core of medical professionalism, tying mind and heart and affirming the importance of the well-being of everyone in the organization. Regarding self-awareness, it is important to ensure that we are aware of our own biases and understand strategies to mitigate these biases. One may consider the attributes of persuasion, conceptualization, and foresight together as one considers the power of a compelling mission and vision as strong motivators for shared action within the organization. Stewardship provides an opportunity to hold individuals accountable for their actions and behavior, establishing policies and practices that are fairly applied.

Remaining committed to the growth of others is key to the sustainability of an inclusive culture, providing a healthy pipeline of future leaders. Moreover, by building community there is an opportunity to exercise consensus-driven, shared decision making.

Based on our experience, we recommend adding cultural humility to this list of attributes. Cultural humility highlights the importance of respecting the lived experiences of others, and determines how best to leverage the array of experiences represented in an organization in sustaining the strengths of the culture of the organization. This is particularly important in healthcare, where cultural differences can impede the reporting of safety and quality concerns. It also reminds us about the potential impact that external forces may have on the culture of the organization, affirming the importance of remaining flexible in strategic planning while also adhering to core values.

As we consider the practical application of inclusive leadership skills in the workplace it is important to recognize the infrastructure and processes that are needed to facilitate the output, and input, of inclusive leaders, while ensuring engagement with the workforce. From an infrastructure perspective, it is helpful to develop a mechanism that provides opportunities for staff to air concerns and ensure open lines of communication with leadership. This can be accomplished by hosting town halls and establishing a network of affinity groups. As one considers processes, transparency is an essential characteristic of an inclusive culture. Establishing clear guidelines for promotion to higher levels in the organization as well as a fair and objective hiring process, are examples of inclusive processes.

Comparison of inclusive leadership with other leadership styles

Based on its inherent differences from other leadership styles, inclusive leadership remains markedly distinct, focusing less on productivity as a protocol and more on authentic identities and participation. This includes, engaging in constructive conflict management, and focusing on diversity as an asset. Most accepted and utilized leadership approaches do not value diversity or embrace diverse solutions and perspectives. In contrast, inclusive leadership often employs a more varied approach wherein staff and students from different disciplines or hierarchal positions demonstrate a true value of diversity.[2]

Using inclusive leadership as a practical solution rather than a theoretical concept supplants the notion that leaders can only be born, suggesting they can also be taught.[5] Praxis then becomes a moral compass, otherwise altering contrasting leadership frameworks to align more cohesively. This asserts that inclusive leadership requires intentional development rather than random sets of suited skills.

Alternate leadership approaches are often accompanied by contradictory communication and hierarchal patterns. Discouraging open communication inhibits empowerment and potentially prevents optimal solutions.[2,3] Conflict management is a part of every leadership approach in some way, but few engage in constructive management as often as inclusive leadership, or with the same intent.

Table 1

Leadership Approach	Attributes	Strengths	Weaknesses
Servant Leadership	• Lead to serve. • Altruistic • Fosters empowerment, growth • Team mindset	• Natural following • Strengthens teams. • Genuinely positive influence	• Balancing self-care • Burnout • Prohibits ego/greed
Democratic Leadership	• Encourages participation/collaboration. • Increased emotional intelligence. • Utilizes coaching leadership	• Creates team culture. • Open communication • Increased engagement	• Slow • Potential tension over disagreements
Autocratic Leadership	• Increased efficiency • Highly controlling • Relies heavily on structure/discipline	• Fast decisions • Clearly defined roles • Streamlined processes	• Poor long-term management • Imbalanced work atmosphere • Lack of diversity
Transformational Leadership	• Long-term planning with clear communication • Purpose-driven • Values growth and development • Creates employee-centric work envrionment	• Involves team, increasing purpose. • Teach to lead. • Rooted in transformative change	• Lacking detail • Lacking accountability • Lacking planning
Transactional Leadership	• Typically, higher-ranking (founder, CEO, etc.) • Performance-oriented • Monitors progress • Communicates about work	• Organized and focused on goals, timelines, etc. • Clearly communicated expectations to meet goals. • Measures progress/performance	• Lack of concern for employee wellbeing • Limited room for growth or development • Disregard for employee input
Laissez-Faire Leadership	• Provides necessary resources to meet goals. • Encourages team to problem, solve, take accountability. • Decreased pressure on production. • Limits input	• Increased employee freedom without interference • Encourages self-management	• Limited/no managerial input • Employee distraction • Decreased productivity
Charismatic Leadership	• Increased communication skills • Persuasive and inspiring • Outcome-driven • Engaging and positive	• Mobilizes groups toward unified goal. • Connects emotionally. • Inspires positive change.	• Potential for burnout • Lack of charisma/passion in group when compared to leader.
Inclusive Leadership	• Listening • Empathy • Healing • Self-Awareness • Persuasion • Conceptualization • Foresight • Stewardship • Commitment to the Growth of People • Building Community[1] • **Cultural Humility**	• Strengthens teams • Builds culture • Creates a platform for accountability • Mobilizes groups towards unified goal	• Takes time to build culture • Will not engage all personality types

Comparative list of leadership skill sets, focusing on key attributes, strengths, and weaknesses

Transformational leadership seeks to empower teams, embracing diversity and the perspectives and resolutions it can bring. However, the approach falls short in focusing on the inclusion of a variety of viewpoints. Inclusive leadership's promotion of a problem-solving environment is reliant on consistently revisiting shared goals, and ensuring all parties are collectively acknowledged and valued in the process; other leadership approaches do not engage in diversity in this way.[6] Inclusive leadership supports increased responsiveness to the opportunities and challenges that diversity can bring. It acknowledges the benefits and value of diversity, creating an innovative and highly productive workforce. Inclusive leadership recognizes the necessity behind the purpose, developing protocols and practices that promote equity alongside diversity and inclusion.[5] It is the commitment to equity and an organizational shift in how diversity is directly addressed that sets inclusive leadership apart from other leadership approaches. See Table 1 to view a comparative list of leadership skill sets.

Measuring the inclusivity of the culture

Most organizations adhere to a data-driven approach for initiatives that embrace the primary business objectives. We have utilized the Diversity Engagement Survey (DES) as a tool to track progress in achieving the goal of inclusive excellence. This tool measures the inclusivity of the culture across eight factors: common purpose, trust, appreciation of individual attributes, sense of belonging, access to opportunity, equitable reward and recognition, cultural competence, and respect.[7] The DES was initially piloted in a single academic center and then expanded to 13 other systems in the United States. It was validated in a cohort of 13,694 participants.[7] An analysis of populations within the cohort demonstrated differences in the responses based on ethnicity and sex.

Our group examined the intersection of professionalism and inclusivity in academic medicine and noted differences in the perceptions of the operationalization of professionalism standards based on sex, ethnicity, and sexual orientation. Notably, individuals from marginalized populations were more likely to express grievances related to judgment regarding their professional behavior in the workplace and were more likely to consider leaving the institution compared to others because of inequities in the application of professionalism standards.[8] The physical well-being of individuals has been demonstrated to also be negatively impacted by the culture of the workplace.[9] These observations underscore the importance of building an inclusive culture to optimize the retention and well-being of all members of the workplace. The DES results are incorporated into a department scorecard shared annually with department chairs that also includes diversity related spending, demographics, and different avenues of outreach.[10]

Strategies to address microaggressions, discriminatory behavior, and bullying in the workplace

Within the fabric of the culture, there are daily interactions between individuals within the workplace that are less than ideal. This behavior may be rooted in unintentional bias, and exacerbated by circumstances such as lack of sleep, hunger, displaced anger, or a feeling of being overwhelmed by tasks and densely packed schedules. The external expression of this tension may be evidenced as a microaggression.

A microaggression may be defined as brief and subtle comments or behaviors that communicate hostile, derogatory, or unwelcoming messages toward others. In many instances, this may be directed toward individuals from underrepresented populations. Discriminatory behavior is defined as the unjust or prejudicial treatment of distinct categories of individuals, especially on the grounds of ancestry, age, or sex.

Another commonly reported behavior is bullying, which is defined as an ongoing and deliberate misuse of power in relationships through repeated verbal, physical, and/or social behavior that intends to cause physical, social, and/or psychological harm.

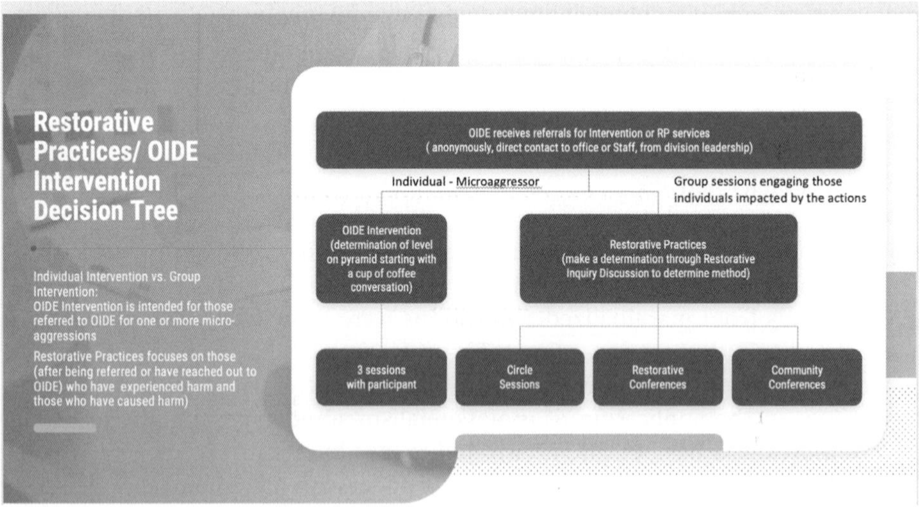

Figure 1: Two prong approach to address discriminatory behavior in the workplace; On the left, note the brief description of an individualized approach and on the right, note the description of the restorative process focused on the unit impacted

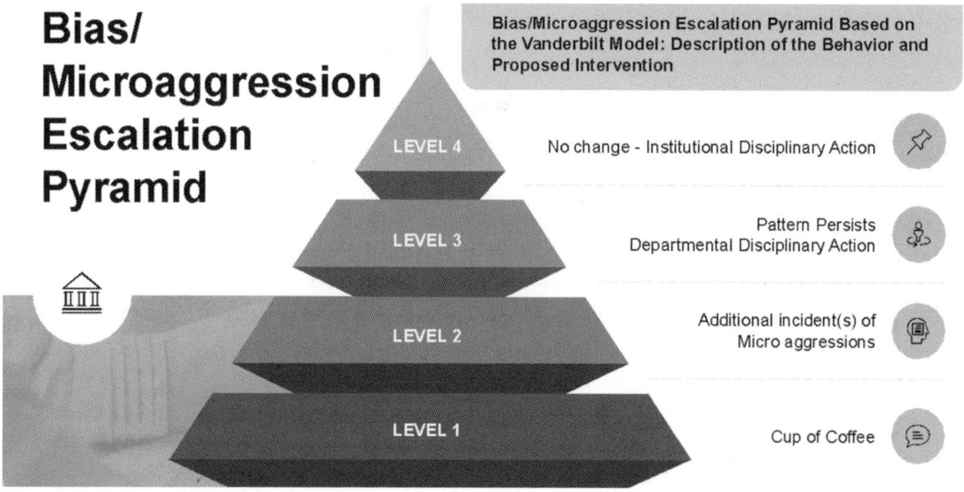

Figure 2: An incremental process is implemented at Level 1 following an initial microaggression; if more persistent instances are observed then subsequent intervention may be necessary

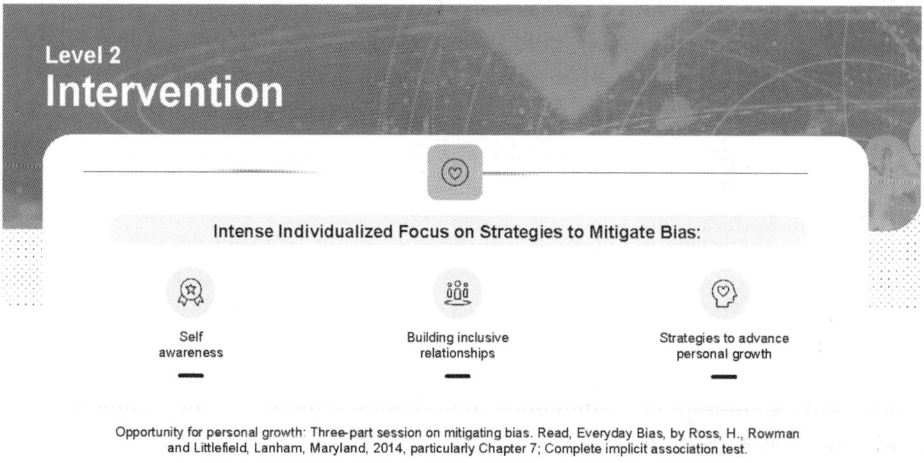

Figure 3: The components of Level 2 are illustrated.

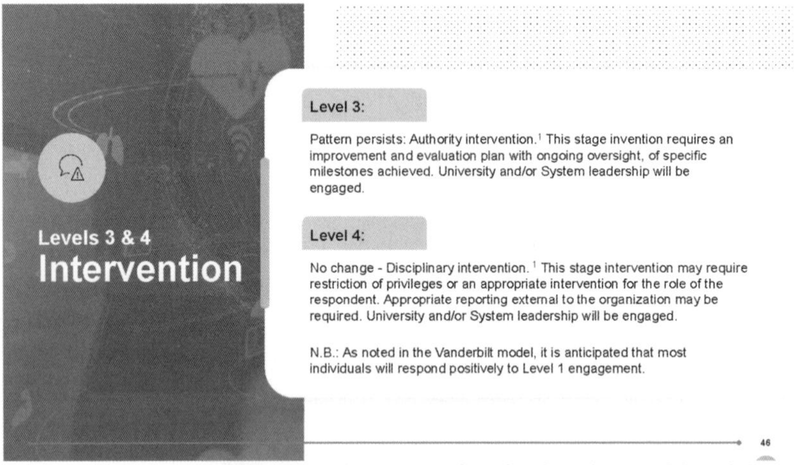

Figure 4: If the interventions have been completed at Levels 1 and 2 and the aggressor continues show patterns of discriminatory behavior, then institutional polices (often driven by Human Resources) will be initiated, as described in this Figure in Levels 3 and 4.

These behaviors and those that may be similarly described require a specific level of attention. The Office of Inclusion, Diversity, and Equity at Penn Medicine developed a process to address the aggressor and those individuals who acutely experienced discriminatory behavior. The former intervention is based on the Vanderbilt model to address professionalism issues and the latter is based on restorative practice. Figure 1 depicts the two processes.

Individual intervention

There are four levels of intervention depending on whether or not this is the first reported incident or if there have been repeated reports (See Figure 2). If this occurrence is the first incident, then there is a peer-to-peer discussion with the aggressor, outlining the complaint, and noting the inappropriate reported behavior. In most instances, this first conversation is sufficient to reduce a repeated incident.

The second level applies to those instances in which the aggressor has had an initial conversation but then repeats the same behavior. This three-session intervention is a one-on-one process that has the primary purpose of developing greater self-awareness, identifying the source of personal bias, and actively developing strategies to mitigate bias (See Figure 3). Repeated instances of discriminatory behavior will require additional disciplinary action (See Figure 4.)

Restorative practice

The integration of restorative practices within the framework of inclusive leadership in medical centers presents a strategic approach to improving relationships and addressing the challenges of diversity and conflict in health care settings. This approach is consistent with the broader concept of inclusive leadership, which is viewed as a strategic response to global and local diversity, emphasizing the management and understanding of diversity in all its dimensions.[11] The adoption of restorative practices in medical centers can greatly benefit inclusive leadership by prioritizing open communication, empathy, understanding, and conflict resolution.[12]

Fostering effective communication

Effective communication is crucial in medical settings to prevent misunderstandings and ensure high-quality patient care. Restorative practices facilitate this by creating safe spaces for dialogue, where concerns and experiences can be openly shared.[13] This approach is supported by inclusive leadership, which values transparency and trust, both of which are essential for fostering a healthy workplace culture.[11]

Building empathy and understanding

Empathy, a fundamental aspect of restorative practices, plays a critical role in health care, as understanding diverse perspectives can lead to improved patient outcomes. Restorative practices encourage individuals to consider the experiences and emotions of others, fostering a culture of empathy and support.[11] This is particularly important in diverse teams, where inclusive leadership aims to ensure that all members feel valued and understood.[11]

Addressing and resolving conflicts

Conflict resolution is a significant benefit of restorative practices in medical centers, offering a structured approach to understanding disputes and repairing relationships.[13] Inclusive leadership leverages these practices to address conflicts constructively, thereby maintaining team effectiveness and high quality patient care.[10]

Promoting continuous learning and growth

Inclusive leadership and restorative practices both emphasize the importance of continuous learning and growth. In the context of medical centers, this extends beyond medical knowledge to include the development of interpersonal skills for working in diverse teams.[12] Restorative practices facilitate reflective learning, enabling teams to learn from conflicts and become stronger as a result.[13] These interventions are important components of building accountability within an inclusive culture.

An effective inclusive leader will need to ensure that everyone understands the impact of their actions and behaviors on the culture of the institution. There should also be greater transparency related to recruitment of new talent, opportunities for professional development, and the fairness of evaluations.

All of these processes should undergo a recurring assessment to ensure objectivity.

References

1. Higginbotham E, Byyny RL. Renewing the commitment to professionalism in the House of Medicine. The Pharos of Alpha Omega Alpha. Summer 2023; 86(3):2-7.

2. Thompson H, Matkin G. The Evolution of Inclusive Leadership Studies: A literature review. J Leadership Education, 2020 July; 19(3): 15–31.

3. Bradley EH. Diversity, Inclusive Leadership, and Health Outcomes. Int J Health Policy Manag. 2020 Jan; 9(7): 266-8.

4. Mind Tool Content Team. Servant Leadership. https://www.mindtools.com/ad648ub/servant-leadership.

5. Rayner S. Educational Diversity and Learning Leadership: A Proposition, Some Principles and a Model of Inclusive Leadership? Educational Review. 2009 Nov; 61(4): 433–7.

6. Ashikali T, Groeneveld S, & Kuipers B. The Role of Inclusive Leadership in Supporting an Inclusive Climate in Diverse Public Sector Teams. Review of Public Personnel Administration. SagePub. 2020; 41(3): 497-519.

7. Person SD, Jordan CG, Allison JJ, Fink Ogawa LM, Castillo-Page L, Conrad S, Nivet MA, Plummer DL. Measuring Diversity and Inclusion in Academic Medicine: The Diversity Engagement Survey. Acad Med. 2015 Dec; 90(12): 1675-83.

8. Alexis DA, Kearney MD, Williams JC, Xu C, Higginbotham EJ, Aysola J. Assessment of Perceptions of Professionalism Among Faculty, Trainees, Staff, and Students in a Large University-Based Health System. JAMA Netw Open. 2020 Nov 2; 3(11): e2021452.

9. Kearney MD, Barg FK, Alexis D, Higginbotham E, Aysola J. Employee Health and Wellness Outcomes Associated With Perceived Discrimination in Academic Medicine: A Qualitative Analysis. JAMA Netw Open. 2022 Jan 4; 5(1): e2145243.

10. Fahl C, Alexis D, Higginbotham EJ, Xu C, Aysola J. Asserting Accountability to Address Diversity: Report Card as a System of Measurement. Health Equity. 2023 Feb 20; 7(1): 116-25.

11. Hollander EP. Inclusive Leadership: The Essential Leader-Follower Relationship New York: Routledge 2009: xix, 263.

12. Costello B, Wachtel J, Wachtel T. The Restorative Practices Handbook for Teachers, Disciplinarians, and Administrators. Bethlehem, PA: International Institute for Restorative Practices; 2009.

13. Zehr H. The little book of restorative justice. Charlotte (NC): Good Books; 2002.

Chapter 7

Professionalism in note documentation: Should OpenNotes exist?

Douglas S. Paauw, MD, MACP; and Jenny Wright, MD

Professionalism is a hard term to define. There are neat and tidy definitions in the dictionary. The Merriam-Webster dictionary defines professionalism as "the conduct, aims, or qualities that characterize or mark a profession or a professional person."[1] If we look to medical societies we find a description from the American College of Physicians and American Board of Internal Medicine (ABIM) and the European Federation of Internal Medicine, who jointly authorized "Medical Professionnalism in the New Millenium: A Physician Charter" in 2002, which describes it as "placing the interests of patients above those of the physician, setting and maintaining standards of competence and integrity, and providing expert advice to society on matters of health.[2] But, these definitions still fail to describe observable behaviors.

Examples of professional behaviors include patient-friendly communication, timely follow-up on the results for laboratory and radiologic studies, and addressing patient questions in a timely manner. There was a time when these were issues that were addressed in the context of a clinic visit or in a letter sent to the patient following a visit. Today, these are often happening in the electronic health record (EHR), which brings us to the OpenNotes era.

OpenNotes may vary somewhat depending on the medical system in which a provider works, but at a minimum we have all been in it since the implementation of components of the 21st Century Cures Act in April 2021.[3] Since then, federal regulations have required that health care systems offer patients access to their health care information in the EHR, including notes, labs and studies. In October 2022, the definition of electronic health information was expanded to include all electronic protected health information, including notes documenting not only face-to-face visits but also telephone care.

Benefits and challenges of OpenNotes

Benefits	Challenges
Improved patient awareness of their health status, medications	Patient frustration or confusion regarding language, results, notifications in the medical record
Ability to share medical records with other providers without the delay of record requests	Not accessible to all patients
Asynchronous requests for appointment scheduling, medication refills	Lack to provider and staff time to address concerns
Facilitate follow up on chronic medical condition	Inaccuracies in the medical records leading to patient concerns

There are many benefits to patients having access to their medical record. This includes increasing their own awareness of their health, and making it easier for patients to share their health information with others. Patient portals also often allow patients to more easily manage their health by allowing for appointment scheduling and communications outside of office hours.

However, not all is good about patient access to their medical record notes. Patients may have difficulty interpreting physician notes or results that are not written in patient-friendly language. Reading negatively worded, or pessimistic opinions in the notes can have a nocebo effect on their health.[4,5] Also, providers and staff are often not provided with protected time to address patient questions coming through patient portals. As such, the impact of the added hours and stress on health care professionals is a large component of burnout.[6]

There is limited evidence to guide us in regard to the patient experience of accessing their medical record. There was a study published in 2019 based on a pilot of OpenNotes at Beth Israel Medical Center, the University of Washington Medical Center and Geisinger Medical Center that began in 2010.[7] Patients who opted into the pilot were surveyed, with a response rate of 22 percent. Of those who responded, 50 percent felt that reading their notes was important. Patients who did not speak English at home were more likely to use the notes to "make the most of their visits", "remember the plan of care", and "prepare for visits"[7] In addition, patients with fewer years of education were more likely to cite note readings as important for "remembering plan of care" and "preparing for visits."[7] Only three percent reported they were confused by their notes, and 11 percent had concerns about privacy.[7] This offers some very encouraging feedback regarding the value of patient access to their medical records.

Some challenges in patient access to their records stems from the fact that physicians and health care systems need to develop new skills and evolve in this new era. For years, physicians have been trained to be thoughtful about verbal communication and body language while caring for patients. Physicians use active listening, respond to emotional cues, and avoid medical terminology. But historically, patient notes were primarily used for provider communication and billing, not as a patient communication tool. OpenNotes requires improved communication skills expanding to include written and digital communication.

Patient sensitive word choice

When relying on written words alone, body language, tone of voice, and overall context of a message can easily be lost or misinterpreted. Many words that are used casually by medical providers, such as complaint, refused or failed can be interpreted as callus by a patient reading them.[8,9] Word choice in the OpenNotes era is extremely important. There are different frameworks that can be used, reflecting on which words could be considered harmful rather than healing and conveying empathy.

Word choices

Harmful words	Healing words
Chronic	Persistent
Complaining	Suffering
Failed	Ineffective

Another framework is to take a patient perspective on language, attempting to predict where there could be misinterpretation.

Language from a patient's perspective[8]

Potential interpretation	Examples
Question patient credibility	Patient ***denies*** fever Patient ***claims*** NSAIDs don't work She ***reports*** a history of "seizure"
Implication that patient is at fault	She ***failed*** chemotherapy He ***insists*** that he cannot exercise to lose weight
Eliciting a stereotype	He is ***vasculopathy*** Patient is ***disheveled***
Difficult patient	Patient ***perseverated*** on her pain Patient ***refused*** statin therapy
Authority	***I stressed the importance*** of diet and exercise
Dismissive	I am ***just*** calling to check on you We have ***done everything we can*** There is ***nothing more we can do***

Expectation setting

There was a time when patient-provider communication was largely limited to clinic visits, or through communication with the clinic during office hours. However, with OpenNotes and patient portals, patients may obtain their lab results as soon as they are entered into the EHR, and patients may be sending their providers messages at any time. It is impossible to predict every expectation a patient may have, but setting some boundaries may be useful to prevent disappointment, and for patient safety.

EHR boundaries

Expectations	Example
Ideal patient portal uses	• Scheduling appointments • Routine refills of medications • Brief focused follow up as negotiated during recent clinic visit
Inappropriate patient portal uses (concern for possibility of unsafe care)	• New symptoms • Requests to start a new medication • For testing or referrals • To fill out paperwork
Explanation of how messages are handled	Hours during which messages are viewed • Timeframe for a response • Team member(s) who may respond on behalf of the physician
Handling of test results	• Timing between when results are released through the portal and if/when the ordering provider comments on those results to the patient

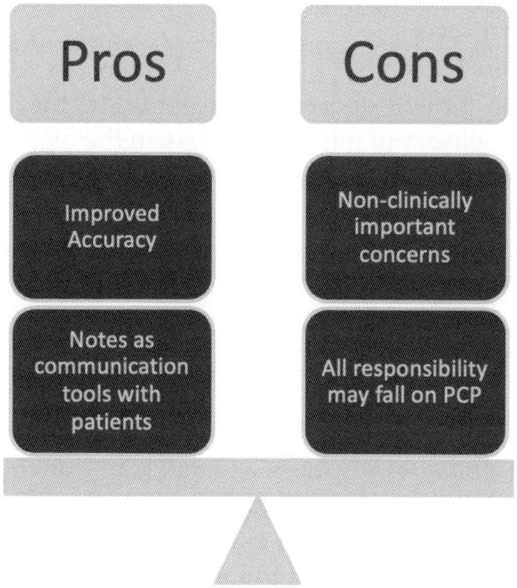

Integrity and accuracy in documentation

OpenNotes can result in patients becoming proof readers, which can have both benefits and challenges. Some of the benefits are that this has the potential to improve notes—offering further reason to curtail inaccurate or out-of-date problem lists and maintain accurate medication lists. Also, patients will potentially see cutting and pasting from previous documentation and other inappropriate documentation practices.

It can be time consuming when patients request that clinically non-important details be changed or clarified. And in many EHRs, though many different providers can edit the problem list, medication list, and other medical history, a patient's request for edits or corrections are likely to all fall on PCP.

Potential for inequity in access to care

Another aspect of medical professionalism that can be problematic with increased dependence of health care systems on the EHR is equity in patient access to care. Many systems are increasingly investing resources into communication through patient portals, and neglecting to maintain and innovate other means of patient communication. Patient use in patient portals is higher in those under 65 years old, with those higher levels of education, and those who live in urban environments.[10] As medical professionals it is critical that we advocate for accessible means for patients and providers to communicate outside of the EHR and patient portals.

Additional considerations

In order for providers to practice professional behaviors within the EHR—timeliness in responding to patient questions and requests, thoughtful use of patient friendly language; and delivery of high quality care in the digital age—we likely need to change what we do. Patient expectation setting is paramount. Patient portal user agreements could be a means of starting this discussion. It is important to acknowledge that these measures will take time to perform and physicians will likely need to advocate for this. And, as more and more care moves to being provided outside of patient visits, in order to keep practices financially solvent, billing for this care will likely be necessary.

An evolution

Professional physician behaviors have, and will continue to, evolve with time. In the current OpenNotes era, a renewed focus on digital communication skills is required, with attention to word choice to convey messages accurately and empathically. Physicians are also going to need to take the lead on advocating for patients with limited access to technology and for protected time for providers and staff to care for patients in this new space.

References

1. Merriam-Webster. Professionalism. https://www.merriam-webster.com/dictionary/professionalism.

2. ABIM Foundation. The Physician Charter. . https://abimfoundation.org/what-we-do/physician-charter#:~:text=Professionalism%20is%20the%20basis%20of,society%20on%20matters%20of%20health

3. U.S. Food and Drug Administration. 21st Century Cures Act. https://www.fda.gov/regulatory-information/selected-amendments-fdc-act/21st-century-cures-act

4. Blease C. Sharing online clinical notes with patients: implications for nocebo effects and health equity. J Med Ethics. 2023; 49: 14–21.

5. Hutchins GPJ, Stone VE, Hall KT. Open notes: Unintended consequences and teachable moments. J Med Ethics. 2023; 49: 28–9.

6. Stillman M. Death by Patient Portal. JAMA. 2023 Jul 18; 330(3): 223-4.

7. Walker J, Leveille S, Bell S et al. OpenNotes After 7 Years: Patient Experiences With Ongoing Access to Their Clinicians' Outpatient Visit Notes. J Med Internet Res 2019 May 6; 21(5): e13876.

8. Epstein AS. Not Just Words. Caring for the Patient by Caring About Language. JAMA Intern Med. May 13, 2013; 173(9): 727-8.

9. Pantilat S. Communicating With Seriously Ill Patients. JAMA, March 25, 2009—Vol 301, No. 12:1279-81.

10. Yang R, Zeng K, Jiang Y. Prevalence, factors, and association of electronic communication use with patient-perceived quality of care from the 2019 Health Information National Trends Survey 5-cycle 3: exploratory study. J Med Internet Res. 2022; 24(2): e27167.

Chapter 8
Hypocrisy in the clinical learning environment

Jay Manoj Brahmbhatt, MD

In the clinical space, medical students often observe professional behavior that is discordant with the standards to which they are held accountable. Medical students are expected to assimilate into the medical profession by aligning with codes of professionalism delineated by medical schools. Students face assessments of their academic competence and communication skills, but also subjective judgments of their behavior, personality, and appearance.[1,2] Students are under constant scrutiny in the shadow of these professional codes, a surveillance of which they are keenly aware.[1]

A clinician educator's role necessitates assessing how a student's performance and behavior measures to prescribed curricular objectives and professionalism milestones. What is a student to think, when that educator fails to exhibit those same professional values?

Hypocrisy refers to behavior that is incongruent with stated values. It can have a profound impact on students, and like other aspects of unprofessionalism, demands attention from the medical education community. Being labeled a hypocrite may feel insulting or evoke frustration. It is necessary to acknowledge the presence of hypocrisy in the clinical learning environment to elicit critical self-reflection in educators and institutions.

Hypocrisy in medicine and psychology

Hypocrisy has not been directly studied in the clinical learning environment or in the context of medical education. However, it is not a novel term in medicine and psychology. There are rich studies of hypocrisy in the field of personality and social psychology.[3] These studies help define hypocrisy as "inconsistency between words and deeds, which people tend to dislike."[4,5] A hypocrite has been defined as one who sends "false signals" or one who "condemns moral failings of other people but behaves badly him- or herself."[4] These definitions are important to consider when building a framework for hypocrisy in medical education.

Hypocrisy is directly mentioned in medical literature within specific contexts of medical culture. Case studies and commentaries recognize hypocrisy in topics such as the practice of defensive medicine to avoid litigation[6,7] in punitive consequences from quality and safety-oriented morbidity and mortality conferences,[8] and in the treatment of health care providers by executives and company leaders of hospitals.[9]

Within the context of medical education literature, there are several widely researched phenomena that are adjacent to hypocrisy. There are studies evaluating students' perceptions of mistreatment,[10] professionalism,[1,11] social support and resiliency,[12] and role models,[13] as well as trust in the clinical learning environment.[14] These are experiences in which medical students face potential conflict in their interface with the clinical learning environment. These conflicts are ubiquitous and formative for medical trainees as they are in the process of assimilating into the professional culture of medicine.

Culture and the hidden curriculum

A medical student's transition during the clinical learning environment can be turbulent. There is a stark difference in the culture of pre-clinical lecture halls and the culture of hospital wards and clinics. The familiarity of lectures and assignments evaporates, questions no longer have multiple choice answers, and evaluations are not a percentage of mistakes and successes. A student's educational experience, previously the sole focus of their classroom environment, becomes an ancillary element of the clinical space, of which the primary purpose is to serve patients.

The culture of the clinical learning environment is a dynamic amalgam of the behaviors, biases, and values of resident physicians, attending physicians, nurses, technicians, patients, patient's families, and the institutions which house them. Through routine engagement, the culture of the clinical learning environment imparts unsanctioned and unstructured lessons to students, a phenomenon that has been referred to as the "hidden curriculum."[15] The hidden curriculum characterizes an important aspect of the socialization of medical students into professional physicians.[15,16]

The hidden curriculum is generally framed as dissonant with the formal curriculum, which is a medical school's published and forthright goals and objectives.[15] While the formal curriculum consists of idealized lessons and objectives to build students into physicians, the hidden curriculum is viewed as the obstacles within a clinical environment that may hinder a student's professional and personal growth.[16-18]

The formal curriculum is intentionally managed by a medical school. In a controlled environment—such as a classroom in which a lesson plan is delivered simultaneously to all students—it is possible to assess the alignment of a course with its curricular goals. Controlling the formal curriculum is a challenge in the clinical setting. As the clinical learning environment is designed for patient care, not formalized education. Students on the same clinical rotation may have drastically different clinical and pathological exposure. Students on a general surgery rotation in the summer may deal with mostly traumas, while students on during other times of the year may see fewer traumas and more infections. The formal curriculum can try to remedy this difference with lessons, but cannot predict or control a student's clinical exposure.

The hidden curriculum may be even more difficult to control. The idealism of a medical school's professionalism curriculum—the standards by which students are to be held and judged—may not always bear true. Ultimately, the people within the clinical learning environment—the people who create its culture and inspire the hidden curriculum—may, or may not, align with the values expected of medical students. Herein lies the potential for hypocrisy.

Domains of hypocrisy

To explore real examples of hypocritical behavior, we held a series of interviews with nine fourth-year medical students from several university-affiliated medical schools around the United States (these interviews are part of a multi-institutional study that is ongoing at the time of writing this chapter). In preliminary analyses, motifs came to light in these interviews that were commonly experienced by students and their peers. One point connected each of these domains: students were left feeling harmed, vulnerable, and disillusioned by their educators and schools. These domains of hypocrisy are described below.

Domain 1: Feedback, evaluations, assessments

Some of the most common points of distress students experience revolve around the process of grading, evaluations, assessments, and receiving feedback. A medical school's curricular objectives or milestones exist to guide a student's growth. They also serve as a tool with which a student's growth may be judged. Much systemwide effort has gone into standardizing this process.[19-21] Excerpt 1 is representative of comments made by all interviewed medical students and expresses the cognitive dissonance experienced by students when that which should be a transparent and standardized process for evaluations and grading becomes opaque and subjective.

Excerpt 1:

> I worked with a few residents every day. I thought they were great. The feedback they gave me was great. I filled out the form with them every day. I was seeing lots of patients, they liked me, I did great.
>
> I spent 80 percent of the time with one person who gave me awesome feedback and then, someone I had never even met, gave me a grade based off of her reading of the [feedback forms] that all said very nice things about me. She just said, "ok, I'll be giving you a high pass..." I understand you're the program director, I understand you're an attending, but you've never interacted with me.

I think a lot of it is arbitrary. I worked really hard... It's so random, you can work really hard and get a bad grade, or you can work not that hard and get a good grade... When it's in my hands, I'm going to give people as high a grade as I possibly can."

The Association of American Medical Colleges (AAMC) has proposed specific guidelines to aid in the assessment of medical students, regarding clinical competencies[19] and professional activities.[20] Similarly, the Accreditation Council for Graduate Medical Education has created exhaustive milestones for each medical specialty to aid in evaluations in graduate medical education.[21] Even in a competency-based grading system, students reflect an inherent sense of subjectiveness, and consequently, a lack of transparency in the evaluation and grading process.

The lack of transparency is an obstacle in learners' ability to trust clinician educators, and by extension, medical schools and health care institutions.[22,23] In interviews done for this chapter and in selected literature, students reported concerns regarding a lack of training for evaluators, their subjectiveness of feedback; the arbitrariness or disjointedness of quantitative grades derived from feedback; and academic hierarchy and fear of retaliation regarding the evaluation process.[24,25]

Domain 2: Clinical knowledge and medical errors

This domain is purposefully broad, encompassing lapses in medical knowledge, and medical and system errors. Students acknowledged that their primary role was that of a learner. Upon entering the clinical learning environment, many felt that they were perceived as lacking authority or legitimacy by supervisors, thereby discounting the years of learning leading to their clinical rotations. This is represented in Excerpt 2.

Students also felt they were expected to demonstrate humility, and to be open to the knowledge imparted on them by superiors for the rest of their careers.

As is represented in Excerpt 3, they also recognized a double standard in which their superiors were not held to the ideal of being lifelong learners, demonstrating humility in the face of mistakes, or demonstrating a willingness to learn and grow.

Excerpt 2:

My second day on my very first rotation and...I [only] knew the [name of the] surgery we were doing. So, I had read up on the surgery and I knew the patient and that was pretty much it... This physician just came in and started... asking me questions that I had never heard of, asking me about surgical techniques and different tools that are used. And if one tool is not available, which one would I use?

One of the residents there, I had met them the day before...asked me a question... about anatomy, which I knew. So, I opened my mouth to answer and that surgeon said, "I wouldn't bother asking her anything. She doesn't know."

Excerpt 3:

I did my whole presentation and came up with my diagnosis and plan, and after all of that, all she said was [that] my definition of dysmenorrhea was wrong, and when I told her what I had learned she said "let's look it up." I had just come off my OB-GYN rotation, so I knew that what I had said was right, and she just said, "I guess we both learned something." Well what did I learn? That I was right?

And then there are... [other attendings] who will just show how to be wrong and do it in a way that has humility. Because, if that's the way I responded when I didn't know something with my attendings, I would get destroyed, they'd hate me.

Everybody's a lifelong learner, until they're not.

Students live in fear of making mistakes,[26,27] whether due to fear of disappointing mentors, looking foolish in front of peers, being ridiculed, or being graded poorly.[28,29] Acts designed to corner or humiliate students, such as asking purposefully complex questions beyond the scope of the learner, have been shown to be ineffective pedagogical tools and are becoming less common. Pimping and belittlement are toxic phenomenon in the clinical learning environment,[28,29] going directly against the necessary humanistic values (e.g., humility, respect, patience) of a clinician-educator.[30]

A disregard or denial of mistakes is an undesirable trait in a learner, one that can be dangerous and lead to medical errors. Students experience distress by the very act of witnessing errors, even those in which they play no role.[31] When errors are not disclosed to patients and students are discouraged from discussing them, distress amplifies.[31] Conversely, students aspired toward those senior physicians who took responsibility for errors. Witnessing such behavior from senior physicians fostered values like honesty and integrity in students.[31]

Lifelong learning is often alluded to as a professional value in medicine,[32] even contributing to long-term professional achievements and career satisfaction.[33] Role modeling humility, and a desire to continuously grow, is indispensable for senior physicians who work with learners. Senior physicians and clinician-educators should be held, at minimum, to the same standard as students: continuously updating clinical knowledge,[30] and welcoming rectification.

Domain 3: Leadership

Leadership and teamwork are critical professional values, and expected skills at all levels from premedical training onward.[19,22,34] Excerpt 4 demonstrates that leadership, while an expected value and skill for medical trainees, is not a guaranteed skill demonstrated by those who are responsible for supervising and evaluating students. Skills relevant to successful leadership, such as emotional intelligence,[35] conflict management, negotiation, or adaptability, are infrequently taught.[36] Excerpt 4 also portrays the consequences and harms experienced when leadership is lacking on a clinical team.

Excerpt 4:

If [the chief resident] spent 10 minutes, it would change this rotation for me... but, instead, anytime I ask a question [they] acted annoyed with me. You're supposed to be the leader of this team but you're not helping me out at all... It's almost harder for you to be doing this. It almost seems intentional, to roll your eyes, to make comments, like when I knocked on the door and told them "I'll be right here when you're ready to leave," and they intentionally left without me...

I felt more nervous or more judged, like was every rotation going to be like this, is everyone this unhappy? This is not what a leader does... You think I'm an idiot and you're right, I don't know anything, I don't know anything about surgery.

The behavior of leaders has been shown to impact residents' job satisfaction, emphasizing an importance of two-way communication and need for specific instructions.[37] The perceptions of the behavior of leaders relates strongly to levels of burnout, professional fulfillment, and attrition among attendings and residents.[38] Residents themselves play an important role in the leadership of clinical teams,[35] taking responsibility for guiding medical students.

Domain 4: Interprofessional teamwork

As described in Domain 3, teamwork is a necessary skill for those working in the medical profession. In interviews, students noted that some of their best role models were those who treated their interprofessional team respectfully. Students knew they would face severe scrutiny for behaving disrespectfully toward any individual. Excerpt 5 illustrates how respectful behavior is not always demonstrated by evaluators, and how disrespectful behavior can be an obstacle for learning, and degrade a student's trust in their educators.

Excerpt 5:

All they would do is complain about the nurses, for every single patient, every single page, every single question, it was impossible for [the nurses] to win or do anything right. If I talked like that about anything... I don't know, it wouldn't go over well.

I know the patients are sick and it's a lot of work for the residents to be answering questions, but, isn't that the point? Isn't that the team? Why don't we spend more time with [nurses]? And I had some of the same questions that the nurses did, and I knew that I just couldn't ask them here.

Physicians are often placed in leadership roles in interdisciplinary health care teams.[39] Power differentials and hierarchy can foster opportunities for interpersonal conflict.[40,41] From the perspective of medical students, the power differential between senior physicians and students is adjacent to the differential between attending physicians and other members of the health care team. Denigration of team members by the leader of that team can be disheartening to students, who may view themselves as potential victims.[41] Furthermore, when potential role models exhibit denigrating behavior, it may be normalized and propagated by students.

Interprofessional conflict can be based on disagreements on patient-related tasks, social representation of professional identity, and structural processes such as workload and support.[39,41] Robust interprofessional education has been shown to improve collaborative behavior.[42]

Domain 5: Empathy

A cruel irony demonstrated in education literature is the importance of empathy as a professional value in medicine,[19,34] and the consistent erosion of empathy in the process of medical training.[43-45] Much like in Domain 4, Excerpt 6 shows how a student witnessed behavior from an attending physician that undermined an empathic approach to patient care. Notably, in Excerpt 6, the student also recognized that the behavior was harmful, regardless of its humorous intent.

Excerpt 6:

> They would send me in to see the patient first. Most of the patients would gush about the attending, I mean, they loved [them] so much and had stories about them going back years and years. Then I'd go in to see the attending and the PA and the nurses would all be in the work room.
>
> I get that they were joking, or it was gallows humor or whatever, but I would hear them say some really disgusting stuff about the patients. It made me feel terrible. Then they would mask it so well when they went into the room.

Both the hidden and formal curricula contain features that exacerbate student distress, and are implicated as factors in the decline of empathy and compassion among medical students.[44,45] Distressing aspects within the hidden curriculum included long work hours and lack of sleep leading to isolation and reduced social support and mistreatment; belittlement; and/or gender-specific discrimination from senior physicians.[45,46] Negative role modeling by superiors also plays a large role in the erosion of compassion and empathy.[47] Distressing aspects of the formal curriculum included insufficient bedside teaching leading to decreased patient interaction, and inadequate exposure or time with role models and attendings.[43,45]

Some skills which are intervenable—mindfulness, reflection, and perspective taking—have been associated with higher compassion, though fixed factors such as sociodemographic traits also play a role in levels of compassion.[48] Historically, studies of empathy levels in medical students often suggest an association with age, sex category, and thereby raising concerns for implicit biases in those studies.[49] Specialty choice has also been shown to impact the level of empathy decline during training.[43] Hearteningly, a meta-analysis of 16 studies demonstrated that interventions to promote empathy were effective.[49]

Domains requiring further inquiry: Systemic and institutional culture

The previous domains have focused on interpersonal interactions. The hidden curriculum evolves from the culture of the clinical learning environment. This culture is inherently influenced by systems and institutions. Values, such as service to communities, making access to medical care and education more equitable, or dedication to a diverse and inclusive working and learning environment are being widely adapted into the mission statement of many medical schools. Between 2007 and 2021, 91 percent of medical schools (n=127) changed their mission statements, and 56 percent (n=77) included diversity language.[50] The correlation between diversity language in mission statements and the execution of diversity-related goals is not widely reported. Further outcomes-based exploration is necessary to better understand how the values of systems and institutions may allow for hypocrisy to manifest.

Disillusionment

Clinician-educators judge students as they are challenged academically in the clinical learning environment. Concurrently, students may judge educators who, within that very environment, strain, bend, and break the professional values extoled by their medical school. Seeing such incongruence between professional or institutional values and the behaviors of professionals and institutions is, unfortunately, commonplace. The Medical School Graduation Questionnaire by AAMC, 55 percent of graduating medical students in 2022 experienced "disconnects between what [is] taught about professional behaviors/attitudes, and what [is] demonstrated by faculty."[51] In response, a sense of punitiveness and weaponization has given professionalism a negative connotation.[52-54]

In studies of undergraduate students, witnessing hypocrisy brings about cognitive dissonance.[43,55,56] The experience of cognitive dissonance is a culprit for a student's cynicism and disillusionment.[56] For medical students, experiencing behaviors from superiors that is incongruent with professional and ethical values can be "a paradoxical and profoundly disorienting experience."[57] These students are more likely to suffer "ethical erosion,"[58] and may experience a loss of idealism, and adopt behaviors that run contrary to the virtues of a good doctor.[55,59] Students experience disillusionment in the face of behaviors that clash with their own professional or personal values.[56,59]

Medical students pay close attention to educators' behaviors and actions, extrapolating the values represented therein.[59] When educators' values conflicted with the students, there was a sense of compromising the students' values and prioritizing the dissonant values of their educators.[59] Over time, these experiences can compound and lead to decay in medical students' confidence in their medical school. In the same referenced AAMC survey, 30.6 percent of graduating students felt neutrally or strongly disagreed that their school had "done a good job fostering and nurturing my development as a person."[51]

Intentionality and critical self-reflection

Intentionality, whether a behavior was done knowingly or wantonly, often drives the perception of hypocrisy. Our interviews demonstrate, though, that the perception of the recipient or observer of a behavior may be a more important factor. A clinician may not intend to behave disparagingly. Their comments regarding other members of an interdisciplinary team might be in jest. That clinician may even view themself as a team player or leader. The consequences of that clinician's behavior, though, is both harmful and incongruent with professional values, regardless of intent.

Medical students recognize behavior in the context of expectations set by their medical school. Students recognize the dire consequences if they were to behave in such a manner. They also recognize that clinicians are responsible for their evaluations. They may doubt if a clinician is aware of the school's expectations or if the clinician would respond graciously to feedback regarding their own behavior. In response, students may question their school's expectations, grading policies, and/or choice in educators.

Students cannot determine the intent of every supervising clinician. Clinicians may not recognize their intent unless they take time to examine their own behavior, balance it with their values and self-image, and assess the impact of their behavior.

Shaping a positive force

The anecdotes in this chapter, directly from medical students, may seem familiar. Generation after generation of clinicians share similar horror stories from medical school and residency. These anecdotes are presented to challenge educators to reconsider the necessity of such experiences.

Rather than passively allowing the hidden curriculum to continue exerting negative influences through these types of behaviors, we must actively shape our clinical culture into a positive force for student development.[15,60] The term hypocrisy is not offered here lightly, and it is not offered disparagingly. This term is offered to awaken compassionate clinicians and educators to the profound impact their words and actions have on students who will inherit and shape future clinical culture.

To consider oneself as hypocritical may bring emotional discomfort. Seeking arguments to justify why a behavior was not hypocrisy per se may ease the ego, but will not ease the harmful consequences of that behavior. Consider intentionality, which is certainly one aspect of hypocrisy. A demeaning comment by an attending can bring pain to a patient and dissonance within a student regardless of humorous or nefarious intent. Clinicians cannot demean a patient and expect students to learn empathy.

Critical self-reflection may reveal one's own moral or behavioral failings. It requires a willingness to view oneself, or one's institution, as fallible, well-intentioned but still susceptible to hypocrisy. The energy exerted in arguing to absolve oneself of hypocrisy subverts the opportunity for growth. Rather, by turning a critical eye toward oneself, educators can recognize their impact and strive to rise above hypocrisy.

Acknowledgments

The quotations included in this chapter are excerpts of interviews that are part of a qualitative, multi-institutional, Institutional Review Board exempted study that is ongoing at time of authoring this chapter. The author of this chapter, Jay Brahmbhatt, MD, is Principal Investigator for this study.

The author wishes to express gratitude for his mentors: Dr. Douglas Paauw (University of Washington), an archetypal role model physician and clinician educator; Dr. Mara Bann (University of Washington); and Dr. Jason Wasserman (Oakland University William Beaumont School of Medicine); and Dr. Kajal Mehta (spouse), Manoj and Rajeshwari Brahmbhatt (parents), and Mansi Brahmbhatt (sister).

The author also acknowledges his collaborators, Dr. Allison Rich (University of Michigan);Dr. Juan Lessing (University of Colorado); Dr. Ben Martin and Dr. Joseph Kerley (University of Virginia), and Dr. Sarah Baker (University of Texas Southwestern).

References

1. Finn G, Garner J, Sawdon M. 'You're judged all the time!' Students' views on professionalism: a multicentre study. Med Educ. 2010; 44(8): 814-25.
2. McLachlan JC, Finn G, Macnaughton J. The conscientiousness index: a novel tool to explore students' professionalism. Acad Med. 2009; 84(5): 559-65.
3. Priolo D, Pelt A, Bauzel RSt, Rubens L, Voisin D, Fointiat V. Three Decades of Research on Induced Hypocrisy: A Meta-Analysis. Pers Soc Psychol Bull. 2019; 45(12): 1681-1701.

4. Jordan JJ, Sommers R, Bloom P, Rand DG. Why Do We Hate Hypocrites? Evidence for a Theory of False Signaling. Psychol Sci. 2017; 28(3): 356-68.
5. Tedeschi JT, Schlenker BR, Bonoma TV. Cognitive dissonance: Private ratiocination or public spectacle? Am Psychol. 1971; 26(8): 685-95.
6. Peterson RM. Hippocrates Versus Hypocrisy: Defending Medicine from Defensive Medicine. Curr Surg. 2005; 62(4): 449-50.
7. O'Connell J, Bryan PB. More Hippocrates, Less Hypocrisy: Early Offers as a Means of Implementing the Institute of Medicine's Recommendations on Malpractice Law. J Law Health. 2000; 15(1): 23-52.
8. Sonnenberg A. Hypocrisy and Tragedy of the Commons. Off J Am Coll Gastroenterol. 2021; 116(8): 1766-7.
9. Byock I. Heroism and Hypocrisy: Seeing Our Reflection with 2020 Vision. J Palliat Med. 2020; 23(11): 1417-8.
10. O'Brien KE, Mechaber AJ, Ledford CH, et al. Perception of Medical Student Mistreatment: Does Specialty Matter? Acad Med. 2022; 97(2): 247-53.
11. Hoobehfekr S, Asghari F, Sayarifard A, Kadivar M, Kashefinejad S. Medical students' perception of professionalism climate in clinical settings. J Med Ethics Hist Med. 2021; 14: 10.
12. Casapulla S, Rodriguez J, Nandyal S, Chavan B. Toward Resilience: Medical Students' Perception of Social Support. J Osteopath Med. 2020; 120(12): 844-54.
13. Tagawa M. Effects of undergraduate medical students' individual attributes on perceptions of encounters with positive and negative role models. BMC Med Educ. 2016; 16: 164.
14. Karp NC, Hauer KE, Sheu L. Trusted to Learn: a Qualitative Study of Clerkship Students' Perspectives on Trust in the Clinical Learning Environment. J Gen Intern Med. 2019; 34(5): 662-8.
15. Lehmann LS, Sulmasy LS, Desai S. Hidden Curricula, Ethics, and Professionalism: Optimizing Clinical Learning Environments in Becoming and Being a Physician: A Position Paper of the American College of Physicians. Ann Intern Med. 2018; 168(7): 506-8.
16. Hafferty FW. Beyond curriculum reform: confronting medicine's hidden curriculum. Acad Med. 1998; 73(4): 403-7.
17. Rabow M, Gargani J, Cooke M. Do As I Say: Curricular Discordance in Medical School End-of-Life Care Education. J Palliat Med. 2007; 10(3): 759-69.
18. Martimianakis MA, Michalec B, Lam J, Cartmill C, Taylor JS, Hafferty FW. Humanism, the Hidden Curriculum, and Educational Reform: A Scoping Review and Thematic Analysis. Acad Med. 2015; 90(11): S5.
19. Association of American Medical Colleges. Recommendations for Clinical Skills Curricula for Undergraduate Medical Education. https://store.aamc.org/recommendations-for-clinical-skills-curricula-for-undergraduate-medical-education-pdf.html.
20. Association of American Medical Colleges. The Core Entrustable Professional Activities (EPAs) for Entering Residency. Summary of the 10-School Pilot, 2014-2021. https://www.aamc.org/about-us/mission-areas/medical-education/cbme/core-epas.

21. Accreditation Counceil for Graduate Medical Education. https://www.acgme.org/milestones/milestones-by-specialty/.
22. Dolan BM, Arnold J, Green MM. Establishing Trust When Assessing Learners: Barriers and Opportunities. Acad Med. 2019; 94(12): 1851-3.
23. Kates MM. Trust Is Transparency: Clarify the Clerkship Grading Scale. Acad Med. 2021; 96(1): 11.
24. Bullock JL, Lai CJ, Lockspeiser T, et al. In Pursuit of Honors: A Multi-Institutional Study of Students' Perceptions of Clerkship Evaluation and Grading. Acad Med. 2019; 94(11S): S48.
25. Nesbitt A, Baird F, Canning B, Griffin A, Sturrock A. Student perception of workplace-based assessment. Clin Teach. 2013; 10(6): 399-404.
26. Rubisch HPK, Blaschke AL, Berberat PO, Fuetterer CS, Haller B, Gartmeier M. Student mistakes and teacher reactions in bedside teaching. Adv Health Sci Educ. 2023; 28(5): 1523-56.
27. Miller E. 2010 Humanism in Medicine Essay Contest: Third Place. Acad Med. 2010; 85(10): 1628.
28. Olasoji HO. Broadening conceptions of medical student mistreatment during clinical teaching: message from a study of "toxic"; phenomenon during bedside teaching. Adv Med Educ Pract. 2018; 9: 483-94.
29. McCarthy CP, McEvoy JW. Pimping in Medical Education: Lacking Evidence and Under Threat. JAMA. 2015; 314(22): 2347-8.
30. Branch WT, Kroenke K, Levinson W. The Clinician-Educator—Present and Future Roles. J Gen Intern Med. 1997; 12(Suppl 2): S1-4.
31. Martinez W, Lo B. Medical students' experiences with medical errors: an analysis of medical student essays. Med Educ. 2008; 42(7): 733-41.
32. Hojat M, Nasca TJ, Erdmann JB, Frisby AJ, Veloski JJ, Gonnella JS. An operational measure of physician lifelong learning: its development, components and preliminary psychometric data. Med Teach. 2003; 25(4): 433-7.
33. Hojat M, Kowitt B, Doria C, Gonnella JS. Career satisfaction and professional accomplishments. Med Educ. 2010; 44(10): 969-76.
34. Association of American Medical Colleges. The Premed Competencies for Entering Medical Students. Students & Residents. Accessed January 21, 2024. https://students-residents.aamc.org/real-stories-demonstrating-premed-competencies/premed-competencies-entering-medical-students.
35. Ward HB. Resident Leadership in the Era of COVID-19: Harnessing Emotional Intelligence. Acad Med. 2020; 95(10): 1521.
36. Berenstain LK, Markowitz SD, Byerly SI. Physician Coaching. Anesthesiol Clin. 2022 ;40(2): 337-48.
37. van der Wal MA, Schönrock-Adema J, Scheele F, Schripsema NR, Jaarsma ADC, Cohen-Schotanus J. Supervisor leadership in relation to resident job satisfaction. BMC Med Educ. 2016; 16(1): 1-7.

38. Mete M, Goldman C, Shanafelt T, Marchalik D. Impact of leadership behaviour on physician well-being, burnout, professional fulfilment and intent to leave: a multicentre cross-sectional survey study. BMJ Open. 2022; 12(6): e057554.
39. Bajwa NM, Bochatay N, Muller-Juge V, et al. Intra versus interprofessional conflicts: implications for conflict management training. J Interprof Care. 2020; 34(2): 259-68.
40. Gergerich E, Boland D, Scott MA. Hierarchies in interprofessional training. J Interprof Care. 2019; 33(5): 528-35.
41. Broukhim M, Yuen F, McDermott H, et al. Interprofessional conflict and conflict management in an educational setting. Med Teach. 2019; 41(4): 408-16.
42. Spaulding EM, Marvel FA, Jacob E, et al. Interprofessional education and collaboration among healthcare students and professionals: a systematic review and call for action. J Interprof Care. 2021; 35(4): 612-21.
43. Newton BW, Barber L, Clardy J, Cleveland E, O'Sullivan P. Is There Hardening of the Heart During Medical School? Acad Med. 2008; 83(3): 244-9.
44. Bandini J, Mitchell C, Epstein-Peterson ZD, et al. Student and Faculty Reflections of the Hidden Curriculum: How Does the Hidden Curriculum Shape Students' Medical Training and Professionalization? Am J Hosp Palliat Med. 2017; 34(1): 57-63.
45. Neumann M, Edelhäuser F, Tauschel D, et al. Empathy Decline and Its Reasons: A Systematic Review of Studies With Medical Students and Residents. Acad Med. 2011; 86(8): 996-1009.
46. Hojat M, Mangione S, Nasca TJ, et al. An empirical study of decline in empathy in medical school. Med Educ. 2004; 38(9): 934-41.
47. Phillips SP, Dalgarno N. Professionalism, professionalization, expertise and compassion: a qualitative study of medical residents. BMC Med Educ. 2017; 17(1): 1-7.
48. Wang CXY, Pavlova A, Boggiss AL, O'Callaghan A, Consedine NS. Predictors of Medical Students' Compassion and Related Constructs: A Systematic Review. Teach Learn Med. 2023 Oct-Dec 35(5):502-13.
49. Fragkos KC, Crampton PES. The Effectiveness of Teaching Clinical Empathy to Medical Students: A Systematic Review and Meta-Analysis of Randomized Controlled Trials. Acad Med. 2020; 95(6): 947-57.
50. Dens Higano J, Tilburt JC, Hafferty FW. Words matter: Tracing the implicit meaning of diversity language (and its absence) in medical school mission statements. J Natl Med Assoc. 2023; 115(1): 18-25.
51. Association of American Medical Colleges. Medical School Graduation Questionnaire: 2022 All Schools Summary Report.; 2022. Accessed March 23, 2023. https://www.aamc.org/media/62006/download.
52. Lee JH. The Weaponization of Medical Professionalism. Acad Med. 2017; 92(5): 579-80.
53. Hafferty FW, O'Brien BC, Tilburt JC. Beyond High-Stakes Testing: Learner Trust, Educational Commodification, and the Loss of Medical School Professionalism. Acad Med. 2020; 95(6): 833-7.

54. Roberts LW. High Road, Low Road: Professionalism, Trust, and Medical Education. Acad Med. 2020; 95(6): 817-8.
55. Lempp H, Seale C. The hidden curriculum in undergraduate medical education: qualitative study of medical students' perceptions of teaching. BMJ. 2004; 329(7469): 770-3.
56. Self DJ, Wolinsky FD, Baldwin DCJ. The effect of teaching medical ethics on medical students' moral reasoning. Acad Med. 1989; 64(12): 755-9.
57. Ginsburg S, Regehr G, Lingard L. To be and not to be: the paradox of the emerging professional stance. Med Educ. 2003; 37(4): 350-7.
58. Feudtner C, Christakis DA, Christakis NA. Do clinical clerks suffer ethical erosion? Students' perceptions of their ethical environment and personal development. Acad Med. 1994; 69(8): 670.
59. Phillips SP, Clarke M. More than an education: the hidden curriculum, professional attitudes and career choice. Med Educ. 2012; 46(9): 887-93.
60. Holmes CL, Harris IB, Schwartz AJ, Regehr G. Harnessing the hidden curriculum: a four-step approach to developing and reinforcing reflective competencies in medical clinical clerkship. Adv Health Sci Educ. 2015; 20(5): 1355-70.

Chapter 9
Supporting professional identity formation in medical trainees

Lynn Buckvar-Keltz, MD; and Barbara Porter, MD, MPH

Unprofessional behavior in medical school is associated with subsequent disciplinary action by a state board for deficiencies in professionalism.[1] A conventional view of professional behavior is that professionalism is seen as a trait, virtue, or attitude; that lapses are character flaws; the absence of unprofessional acts is evidence of professionalism; and the presence of unprofessional acts means the trainee or physician is unsuited for the profession. However, a more developmental view is that professionalism is a dynamic evolving process; that lapses happen to everyone and have many causes; professionalism is demonstrated in every clinical situation; and that supportive systems and a professional culture lead to trainees who are professional.

At NYU Grossman School of Medicine the curriculum focuses on professional identity formation (PIF) because there is a direct connection between one's professional identity and their professional behavior. Students are engaged in activities that provide insight into professional identity and moral reasoning using writing, feedback, self reflection, case discussion, and coaching. There are explicit discussions about how PIF fits in with a student's overall identity, and we discuss what professional behaviors are expected in medical students.

There are several objectives of the undergraduate medical education (UME) curriculum:

- Providing a framework and language for medical students to understand their professional identity and professional behavior;
- Articulating the nature of medical professionalism, medicine's social contract, and the values held by physicians;
- Describing the process of professional identity formation and socialization
- Recognizing challenges of merging personal identity with emerging professional identity;
- Understanding the use of professional identity essays (PIE) to help professional identity formation;
- Discussing ethical challenges experienced by clinical medical students and discuss options for facing these challenges;

- Reflecting on stressors that might inhibit professional growth, and
- Reflecting on strategies to support professional growth. A shared mental model of PIF that describes the early adult stage (stage 2) as one in which the individual is mainly focused on themselves, including their individual performance and achievement. In stage 3, individuals are more team-oriented, and establish social norms by checking in with others, and adopting the values of others around them. In stage 4 individuals are integrated professionals who have a discerning principled identity, are centered and able to attend to, and be tolerant of, complexity. These individuals can manage competing values and handle ambiguity. Of note, only a minority of adults are thought to achieve a stage 4 identity.

Conceptual model of professional identity formation

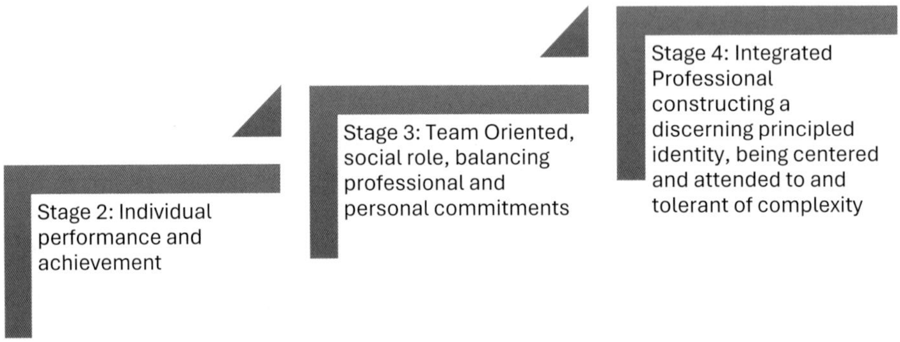

In order to support students' PIF they are required to complete PIEs three times during medical school—at first year orientation, at the end of the preclinical curriculum, and late in the final year of medical school, as a formative tool for growth. The essays are responses to a series of nine written prompts, and have been validated in multiple learners. The essays are evaluated and scored by trained experts. Students receive detailed reports that explain what stage of PIF they are in, with supporting evidence from their responses, and questions to help them reflect and develop insight for their professional growth. The reports also reinforce the language regarding PIF. Students receive confidential reports, and are tasked with writing a reflection on the reports. No faculty or staff see the reports or reflections, but students are encouraged to discuss them with their faculty advisors or other trusted faculty.

Additional activities include lectures in the pre-clinical stage of the curriculum, a case-based workshop on professional behavior challenges in clinical rotations during orientation to clerkships, and a workshop during transition to residency week. This final workshop's objectives are to have students anticipate challenges to their professional identity and professional behavior during internship and to consider options when confronted with situations in which professional values are in conflict.

The professionalism curriculum is intended to also give students the language and grounding to work through professional behavior challenges and challenges to their professional identity during medical school, especially during clinical rotations. Positive role models reinforce PIF, but negative experiences also occur and this curriculum is meant to help students navigate these times. In addition, faculty advisors meet regularly with assigned student mentees throughout medical school and encourage students to share their professional identity formation.

Research on individual student's (n=200 students) PIEs over time show that throughout medical school 47 percent of students' PIF stage increases; 45 percent of students' PIF remains stable; and 7.5 percent PIF stage decreased.[2]

Supporting the professional growth of internal medicine residents

Typically, more than 20 percent of trainees who match into an NYU program come from NYU Grossman School of Medicine, and thus, in recent years have participated in the school's professional identity curriculum. Most of the residency graduates (~48 percent) pursue further training immediately following residency, while the remainder complete a chief resident year (18 percent), become hospitalists (25 percent), or pursue careers in ambulatory medicine (seven percent).

Coaching

Since 2020, NYU internal medicine interns have participated in a coaching program funded by an American Medical Association Reimagining Residency grant. The NYU Transition to Residency Advantage (TRA) program was proposed as a learner-centered program of support from match day through the transition to residency. Recognizing that transitions are vulnerable times for trainees, and that residency requires new skills of regulating one's own learning, integrating a new professional identity, and balancing personal demands, a coaching program was developed to encourage self-directed learning, and a drive toward autonomy.

While all NYU interns were enrolled in the coaching program, NYU Grossman SOM graduates met their TRA coach before the start of intern year, in a meeting with their UME advisor, in order to establish a coaching relationship that bridges the transition to residency. All interns then meet with their coaches four times a year, using reflective exercises to support goal development.

Insights from the experience, thus far, include the observation that with coaching, trainees set higher quality goals than other medical students. These goals are often goals for reflective practice, career development, and scholarship, compared to medical students' goals which are more likely to be general patient care goals.[3]

Additionally, qualitative analysis of focus groups with coaches and coaches support the notion that coaching creates an explicit curriculum for professional growth from medical student to resident, and supports autonomy and self-directed learning, key components of professional identity formation.[4]

Learning communities

Since 2015, the Medicine residency at NYU has used block scheduling as a way to separate inpatient and outpatient time, thereby abolishing the conflict that arises when residents attend clinic while on inpatient wards. Block scheduling enables a weekly academic half-day during outpatient time, and as a result the same cohort of PGY2 and PGY3 residents (1/3 of each class) are together regularly for discussion, conferences, and workshops.

An important component of the academic time is a discussion group that meets the first week of the block, with the same group of seven to eight peers and a consistent faculty member. Over two years, these peer groups meet 16-17 times, and share reflections on topics such as balancing inner terror with outer control, responding to loss, understanding empathy and compassion, gratitude, and other relevant topics. We have observed how resident reflections change over two years, reflecting development in professional identity. For example, early PGY2s are more likely to focus on societal and professional ideals, while late PGY3s more discerning, and tolerant of the complexity of daily work.

Next steps are to study how professional identity changes over three years of residency. Will explicit education on PIF impact professional identity development in residents? What will the progression of professional identity in NYUGSOM educated IM residents look like compared to non-NYU educated peers?

PIF is an ongoing process of development for NYUGSOM students, NYU residents, and faculty.

References:

1. Papadakis MA, Hodgson CS, Teherani A, Kohatsu ND. Unprofessional behavior in medical school is associated with subsequent disciplinary action by a state medical board. J Medical Regulation. 2004; 90(1): 16-23.

2. Lusk P, Ark T, Crowe R, Monson V, et al. Measuring the development of a medical professional identity through medical school. Medical Teacher, Nov 2023; 665-71.

3. Winkel AF, Chang LY, McGlone P, Gillespie C, et al. SMARTer goalsetting: a pilot innovation for coaches during the transition to residency. Acad Med. 2023 May 1; 98(5): 585-9.

4. Park A, Gillespie C, Triola M, Buckvar-Keltz L, et al. Scaffolding the Transition to Residency: A Qualitative Study of Coach and Resident Perspectives. Acad Med. 2024 Jan 1; 99(1): 91-7.

Chapter 10

Medical professionalism in an evolving landscape

Antoinette Pusateri, MD; Hareen Seerha; Sheryl A. Pfeil, MD; and Douglas S. Paauw, MD, MACP

Disclaimer: This manuscript represents the thoughts and opinions of the four authors, unless cited otherwise. "We" is used to refer to thoughts all authors have collectively discussed and agree on.

Medical professionalism in an evolving landscape: what imagery comes to mind when you consider this? Through the lenses of physicians in academic medicine today, there is an overwhelming scene to behold: injustice and discord caused by the COVID-19 pandemic, systemic racism, and war, juxtaposed with the advancements in technology creating new opportunities for health equity and unity. As physicians, we must unite for the health and safety of patients and communities. This vision can only be built on the stable foundation of each physician's professional and personal identity formation. In a system that incentivizes product generation, stress lies in the distance between expectations and realities. By defining the expectations and realities of our lives as physicians in academic medicine, we can leverage advances in technology to bring these lines together, such that our professional identities incorporate productivity, compassion, and fulfillment, in service to our patients, colleagues, and selves.

Bridging the Distance Between Expectations and Reality through Technology

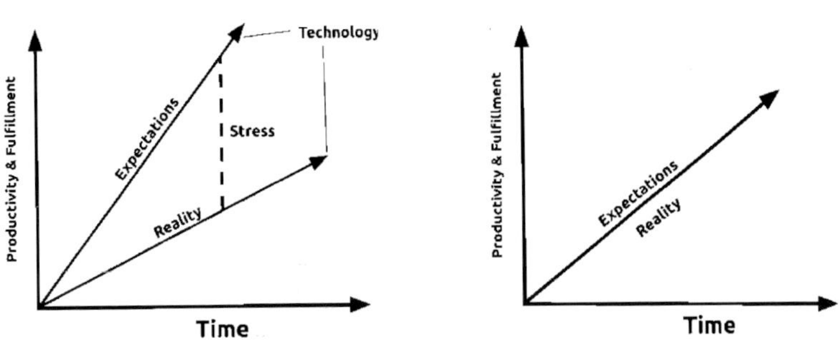

Visual representation of stress burden as reality cannot match the increasing societal and individual expectations of productivity and fulfillment.

Theory that technology bridges this gap, and, therefore, can decrease stress; thus bridging societal and individual expectations within reality.

Background: Health care technology and burnout

Navigating modern technology while maintaining professionalism and competency is often a double-edged sword. However, technology has already become a part of medical practice, whether desired or not. This begs the question: how can technology be used in a way that the benefits outweigh the drawbacks?

Framework for Utilizing Technology in Healthcare

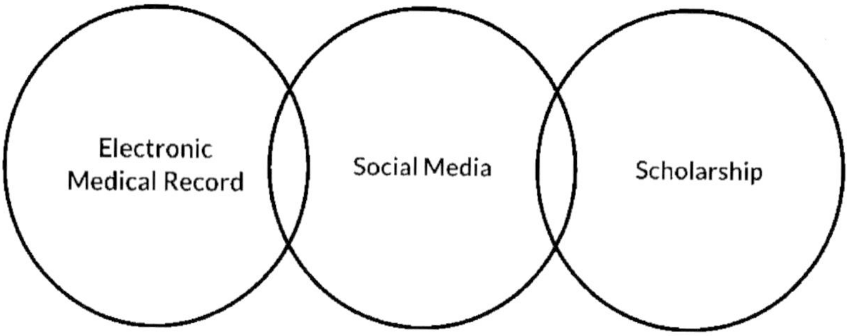

Each modality is interconnected, i.e., patients may reach out to providers via social media, or social media can be used for scholarship.

Burnout is a systemic problem. Causes include inadequate support, more demanding workloads, administrative burdens, underfunded public health infrastructure, and moral injury from being unable to provide the care patients need and providers want to give.[1] Burnout is about a fundamental disconnect between health workers and the mission to serve that motivates them.[2] This manifests in the individual as compassion fatigue. Compassion fatigue is defined as the "convergence of traumatic stress and cumulative burnout." [3]Its physical signs and symptoms include fatigue, irritability, increased negative coping behaviors, lessened empathy, diminished work satisfaction, and an impaired ability to make decisions and care for patients.[3] As such, compassion fatigue directly diminishes both professionalism and competency.[3]

Advancements in technology may feel like something that hastens, not heals, compassion fatigue. In 1950, it was expected that the amount of knowledge a medical student would learn during four years of medical school would double within 50 years; in 2020, this became 73 days.[4] With ChatGPT's advent, admissions committees and academics are navigating how to determine if papers are written by applicants or via artificial intelligence (AI).[5] Also, with the pervasiveness of social media, navigating professional versus personal identities seems harder than ever before. With these advances, and the increasing demands placed on trainees and physicians, technology can make things feel hopeless.

Technology is here to stay, and physicians can use these advances to bridge the gaps in professionalism and competency caused by compassion fatigue.

The expectations of medical professionalism

Defining and understanding professionalism is complex. Medical professionalism has been defined as a social contract between society and the institution of medicine. Society expects that the institution of medicine delivers health care services with expertise, altruism, integrity, transparency, and accountability. The institution of medicine expects physicians to conduct themselves with honesty, respect, and self-regulation, giving them the autonomy for scientific innovation.[6] But, where does the individual physician and their professional and personal identity formation fit into these expectations? Who asks the individual physician what they expect of themselves and of the system? The reality is that individual physicians are expected to adapt, advance, and be ever-present in a world where so many request their presence, without time for proper prioritization and reflection. This can lead to feelings of inauthenticity and inadequacy, the questioning of ability and purpose, all of which are the antithesis of fulfillment, and can lead to further compassion fatigue.

The idea of professionalism can be used as a tool for control; a predetermined script for the socialization of trainees and providers to fit an antiquated model of how physicians ought to be, instead of inspiring an imagination for who physicians should hope to be.[7] Professionalism is as much an individual's responsibility as it is how society perceives the individual.

An example of this social contract in action was illustrated in 2020 when the *Journal of Vascular Surgeons* published an article (now retracted) entitled, "Prevalence of unprofessional social media content among young vascular surgeons."[8] The intention, one author wrote, "was to empower surgeons to be aware and then personally decide what may be easily available for patients and colleagues to see about us," since up to 40 percent of patients search for a doctor online. However, by suggesting that photos where female vascular surgeons were attired in bikinis or swimwear were unprofessional, there was a backlash on social media from health professionals. Many felt such content was unfairly targeting women in medicine, who could, as one female physician wrote, "wear swimwear to the beach in my free time and be a competent and compassionate physician at work," prompting what is known as the "#medbikini" response worldwide.[9] Such a movement emphasizes the mindful approach physicians must take when discussing professional and personal identity formation and societal responsibility; it also demonstrates the intersectionality between professionalism, technology, and social media.

The Institute of Medicine has long advocated that physicians meet patients where they are, in order to provide patient-centered, safe, effective, timely, efficient, and equitable care.[10] Since the COVID-19 pandemic, social distancing transformed the way people interact and get their information, meeting patients and colleagues where they are. This means connecting online via telecommunications, social media, and digital scholarship. The positives and negatives of these technological advances must be evaluated and leveraged for the benefit of patients, colleagues, and all health care providers.

Advances in technology: Electronic medical record (EMR)

The ability for immediate correspondence between patients and physicians through cell phones and apps, including electronic medical record-based instant messaging can be lifesaving and advance the mission of timely and efficient care. Through E-mail and other collaborative online services, medical research, quality improvement, and education efforts can come to fruition by physician teams from

EMR Pros and Cons

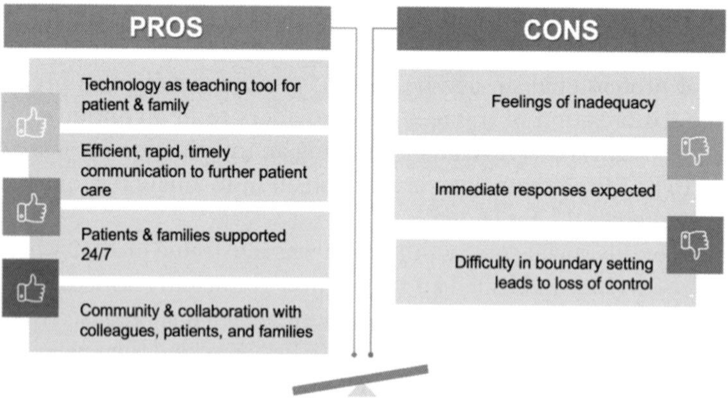

across the hall to across the world. While such telecommunications can connect, elevate, and amplify voices for good, these voices can also inundate physicians. They can prevent them from being present in the moment and blur the lines between professional and personal domains.

Physician productivity has come to be measured by the generation of relative value units (RVU), which allows the system to bundle the time and intensity of the physician's work into a reimbursable cost of care.[11,12] Like every human, the physician's time is finite. In an age where access to the physician is infinite, the system must bridge this obvious disparity by protecting the time of the physician and reimbursing for it accordingly. Primary care physicians spend an average of 52 minutes on workdays managing their EMR inbox, with an additional 19 minutes spent outside normal work hours.[13] It takes the average physician approximately two to three minutes to respond to a single inbox message.[14] Ideally, time would be allocated in the workday to answer patient messages, or the messages would be treated as actual patient visits and be measured as productivity allowing a finite physician workload. Some physicians feel if a patient portal message is greater than 100 words, it constitutes the same time and energy as a patient visit.[15]

Unfortunately, the technology for patient portals developed more quickly than policies that address the time and stress on physicians. Some aspects of messaging are very helpful, such as getting feedback on the effect of recent blood pressure or blood glucose therapy changes or messages to schedule an appointment. Messages such as these can be managed by other members of the care team—medical assistants or nurses—and can help make care more efficient for patients while also reducing the stress placed on physicians.[14] Many institutions have started to charge for patient portal messages including new medical issues or completion of forms, respecting physicians' time and encouraging appropriate assessment for the patient.[16]

Physicians and educators carry a responsibility to not only make sure patients are equipped with enough knowledge to empower themselves between appointments, but to also help patients understand when messaging versus appointments are appropriate. In addition, physicians carry a responsibility to understand how to prioritize messages in the inbox by responding to the most urgent things first. As physicians navigate changes with technology, it is vital that physicians play a larger role in discussing policies around the use of the EMR modifications.

Advances in technology: Social media

In a similar way, social media platforms such as X (formerly Twitter), Instagram, TikTok, Facebook and others allow rapid access to and dissemination of information. Physicians' posts can contribute directly to health care policy and advocacy and demystify medicine for patients or those aspiring to be physicians. Once again, blurred lines between the professional and personal domains of physicians' lives and the reduction of their lives to a series of photos or tweets, can lead to false

Social Media Pros and Cons

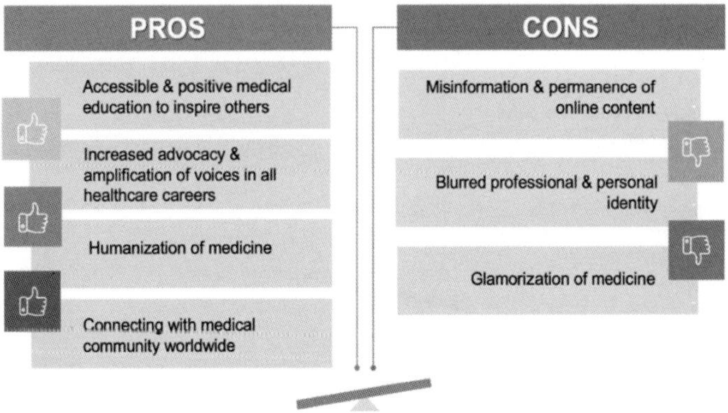

representations of what physicians' lives are or ought to be. Social media accounts can provide physicians a sense of control of their own narrative not often afforded to them in their training or schedule. However, if they lose sight of their purpose in the social media platform, others' expectations of their narratives can ultimately control physicians.

In his book, "Empower Yourself," Harvey Coleman, presents the PIE (performance, image, exposure) theory of success as the primary method for career progression.[17] It postulates that performance, image, and exposure work together to allow for career progression: performance makes up 10 percent of the pie, while image is 30 percent and exposure is 60 percent. Social media can contribute to career progression and even compassion fatigue mitigation through the image and exposure pieces of PIE.

However, no amount of image and exposure can absolve the success and reputation of institutions or physicians who repeatedly, or worse, intentionally, do not practice according to standards. Safe, honest, evidenced-based, patient-centered care is still the standard for success, and is what all human beings deserve.[18] Assuming operation by the standards of care for institutions, exposure via social media can amplify their mission, foster alliances with marginalized organizations, and attract more patients.

The same is true for the individual physician and even trainees: social media can help them control their own narrative in-person and online by defining and promoting their professional career or niche, fostering connections with patients and colleagues across the world, and creating a platform for health policy and

Scholarship Pros and Cons

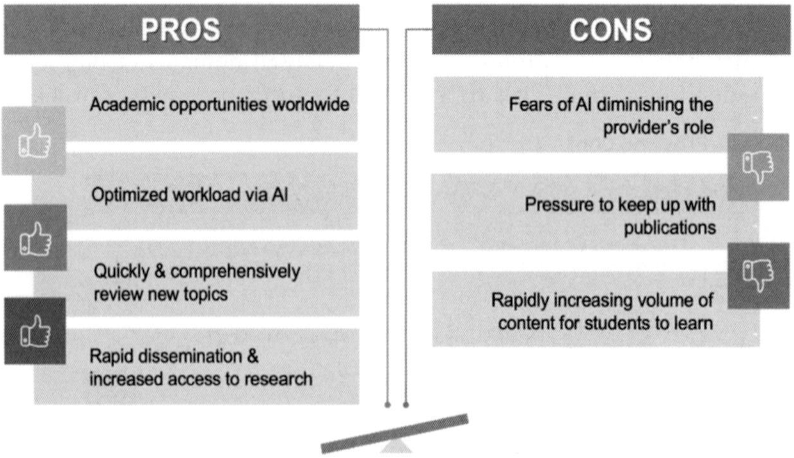

advocacy. Institutions are acknowledging the role of social media in academic visibility and community engagement by integrating such contributions as significant and meritorious for faculty promotion.[19] Therefore, it is important for institutions to consider how social media can be leveraged to engage and educate communities, enhance access to health care, and empower physicians to take control of their narratives in an authentic and constructive way.

Advances in technology: Scholarship

The instant access to the latest research through search engines from Google to PubMed, and the digitalization of medical texts from university health science libraries, helps physicians make in-the-moment, evidence-based decisions for patients. However, the rapid publication of scientific innovations can be hard to keep up with, particularly for trainees still working to learn the foundational principles of medicine. This can contribute to feelings of inadequacy and imposter syndrome for physicians, and widespread confusion and mistrust if such information is released to the public prematurely or incompletely.

Practical Resources for Patient Care

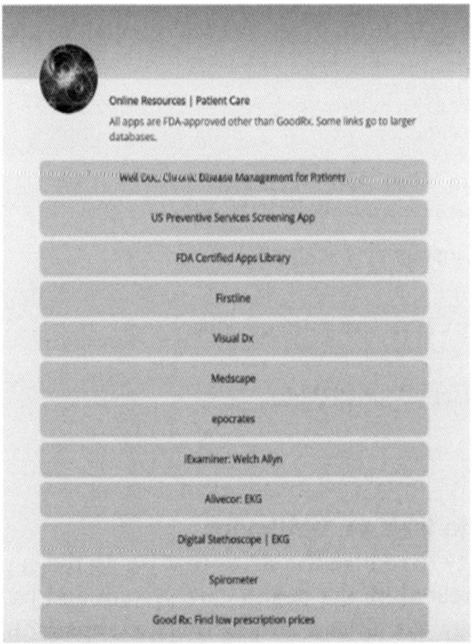

bit.ly/m/MedicalResources

In a similar vein, the innovation of artificial intelligence (AI) in recent years has created opportunities for workload optimization and data processing to help physicians with patient care, research, and education. For example, Epic EMR recently unveiled a new AI-powered system that automatically creates notes from listening to in-office and telehealth patient visits. Hospital systems feel that this will allow for a more organic, focused conversation between physician and patient, enhancing the therapeutic relationship and documentation efficiency.[20]

The advancements in AI have many concerned that it will slowly overtake the physician's role in the future, leading to further thoughts of inadequacy, loss of control, and fear. As OBGYN Richard Paulson writes, "if we measure the 'intelligence' in AI by data regurgitation, passing examinations, and pattern recognition, then perhaps we need to reassess our definitions of what it means to be human, the complexity of the science and art that it takes to be a physician, and adapt these systems to help humankind."[21] Professors at Korea University conducted a national survey to develop core competencies for medical students to define the use of AI in medical education and clinical practice.[22] The Association of American Medical Colleges (AAMC) hosted a webinar series throughout 2024 to discuss the concepts, concerns, equity and ethics of AI in medical education.[23] In a similar way, physicians worldwide should come together to control the narrative of AI in medicine by defining how AI should be used and taught throughout medical specialties and medical schools.

Practical Resources for the Physician

- Communications: Doximity, Zoom, WhatsApp, Microsoft Teams, Google Translate
- Social Media Platforms: Tik Tok, Instagram, Facebook, X (formerly twitter), Threads
- Social Media Management Tools: Canva, Grammarly, Adobe Spark, Content Calendar
- Scholarship: OneNote, Audible, Libby, Journal Club, Choosing Wisely, Visual Dx

Conclusion: Leveraging technology to lead to fulfillment

How can physicians leverage technology to reduce the stress that lies in the gap between the expectations and realities created by the health care system and patients? How can physicians use technology to cultivate productivity, compassion, and fulfillment? Medical professionalism is rooted in authenticity and competency.

Thus, on a systems level, physicians must call for health care institutions to protect time for their professional and personal identity development, including space for self-reflection and mentorship. Physicians must also demand a seat at the table of those meetings institutionally, and nationally, that are adapting or innovating new technologies that will directly impact their work in caring for patients, and be used by physicians including electronic medical records and AI.

Physician organizations such as AΩA are perfectly poised to make this vision a reality as it represents all training levels and all specialties. "To be worthy to serve the suffering" means we must recognize that our own colleagues are suffering. Together, anchored in our commitment to authenticity and competency, we can inspire each other to stay curious and resilient, and provide team-based, patient-centered care.

Taking care of ourselves, writing our narratives, and reminding ourselves of why we chose to be in this miraculous profession, is a small act of rebellion against broader systems. Using technology to our benefit, while acknowledging, learning from, and modifying its drawbacks are all ways to cultivate lasting change to reduce compassion fatigue, and increase competence and professionalism in the trainee and provider.

References

1. Izdebski Z, Kozakiewicz A, Bialorudzki M, Dec-Pietrowska J, Mazur J. Occupational Burnout in Healthcare Workers, Stress and Other Symptoms of Work Overload during the COVID-19 Pandemic in Poland. Int J Environ Res Public Health. Jan 30 2023; 20(3): 2428.
2. De Hert S. Burnout in Healthcare Workers: Prevalence, Impact and Preventative Strategies. Local Reg Anesth. 2020; 13(1178-7112 (Print)): 171-183.
3. Cocker F, Joss N. Compassion Fatigue among Healthcare, Emergency and Community Service Workers: A Systematic Review. Int J Environ Res Public Health. Jun 22 2016; 13(6): 618.
4. Densen P. Challenges and opportunities facing medical education. Trans Am Clin Climatol Assoc. 2011; 122(0065-7778 (Print)): 48-58.
5. Boyle P. Will chatbots help or hamper medical education? Here is what humans (and chatbots) say. AAMC News. https://www.aamc.org/news/will-chatbots-help-or-hamper-medical-education-here-what-humans-and-chatbots-say.
6. Cruess SR, Cruess RL. Professionalism and Medicine's Social Contract with Society. Virtual Mentor. Apr 1 2004; 6(4): 185-8. 4
7. Maristany D, Hauer KE, Leep Hunderfund AN, et al. The Problem and Power of Professionalism: A Critical Analysis of Medical Students' and Residents' Perspectives and Experiences of Professionalism. Acad Med. Nov 1 2023; 98(11S): S32-S41.
8. Hardouin S, Cheng TW, Mitchell EL, et al. RETRACTED: Prevalence of unprofessional social media content among young vascular surgeons. Elsevier; 2020.

9. Johnson LM, Ebrahimgi A. A medical journal apologized after an article prompted health professionals to post images of themselves in bikinis. CNN. July 25, 2020. https://www.cnn.com/2020/07/25/cnn10/medbikini-backlash-and-apologies-trnd/index.html.
10. Institute of Medicine. Committee on Quality of Health Care in America. Crossing the Quality Chasm: A New Health System for the 21st Century. Washington (DC): National Academics Press. 2001.
11. AMA CPT® International. Relative Value Units. https://cpt-international.ama-assn.org/relative-value-units.
12. Nurok M, Gewertz B. Relative Value Units and the Measurement of Physician Performance. JAMA. Sep 24 2019; 322(12): 1139-40.
13. Akbar F, Mark G, Warton EM, et al. Physicians' electronic inbox work patterns and factors associated with high inbox work duration. J Am Med Inform Assoc. Apr 23 2021; 28(5): 923-30.
14. Kummervold PE, Johnsen J-AK. Physician response time when communicating with patients over the Internet. J Med Internet Research. 2011; 13(4): e1583.
15. Berg S. What doctors wish patients knew about using a patient portal. American Medical Association. https://www.ama-assn.org/practice-management/digital/what-doctors-wish-patients-knew-about-using-patient-portal.
16. Diaz N. What 3 health systems are charging for MyChart messages. Becker's Hospital Review. https://www.beckershospitalreview.com/ehrs/what-3-health-systems-are-charging-for-mychart-messages.html.
17. Coleman HJ. Empowering yourself: the organizational game revealed. Bloomington (IN): AuthorHouse; 2010.
18. Institute of Medicine. Committee on Quality of Health Care in America. To Err is Human: Building a Safer Health System. Washington (DC): National Academics Press. 2000.
19. Fitzgerald JJ, Losee JE, Roth RN, Pettigrew C, Thamman R. A Worksheet to Quantify Social and Digital Media Content as Scholarly Products for Academic Promotion. Acad Med. April; 99(4): 404-7.
20. Diaz N. Epic makes AI-powered clinical documentation widely available. Becker's Hospital Review. https://www.beckershospitalreview.com/ehrs/epic-makes-ai-powered-clinical-documentation-widely-available.html?utm_campaign=bhr&utm_source=website&utm_content=latestarticles.
21. Paulson RJ. Artificial intelligence in medicine: it is neither new, nor frightening. F&S Reports. 2023; 4(3): 239-40.
22. Lee YM, Kim S, Lee YH, et al. Defining Medical AI Competencies for Medical School Graduates: Outcomes of a Delphi Survey and Medical Student/Educator Questionnaire of South Korean Medical Schools. Acad Med. Dec 28 2023; 10: 1097.
23. Association of Academic Medical Centers. Artificial Intelligence (AI) in Academic Medicine Webinar Series. https://www.aamc.org/about-us/mission-areas/medical-education/artificial-intelligence-ai-academic-medicine-webinar-series

Chapter 11

Using technology innovation and strategy to combat burnout

Bryan Hendrickson, MD; Peter Georginis, MD; Kevin Smith, MD; Simone Maxey, MHSA; Kevin Pearlman, MD; Sachin Shah, MD; Cheng-Kai Kao, MD; and Bree Andrews, MD, MPH

The current state of well-being includes an awareness of the systemic nature of well-being at the workplace. Life balance is an area of focus; however, there can be an emphasis on "making it fit on your own time" for providers. Medicine may be in a stage of over-reliance on personal factors as it begins to shift focus on systemic interventions.

The future of well-being includes organizations and health systems working broadly to reduce distress and promote well-being. Clinicians are imperfect and organizations can promote limits and supports that boost overall flexibility and integration at work.

Big and small ideas

As health systems move toward wellness there has been a focus on big ideas, such as culture of wellness and efficiency of practice complementing personal resilience leading to professional fulfillment.[1] A culture of wellness is the organizational values and actions that promote personal and professional growth, and compassion for self, colleagues, and patients. Efficiency of practice is the seamless way we work in clinical, educational, and research spheres. Professional fulfillment is happiness, meaningfulness, self-efficacy, and satisfaction at work, and the building of a professional identity.

Within these domains there are slightly smaller ideas. A culture of wellness includes leadership, values alignment, professional development, collegiality, gratitude, flexibility, and managing post-pandemic expectations. Efficiency of practice includes electronic health record (EHR) usability, efficiency, and workload; scheduling work-day, call, and patients; call center, and patient portals; team-based care; reasonable turnaround times; appropriate staffing and teaching; and innovation in practice. Personal resilience includes self-care and compassion, meaning in work, work-life integration, cognitive and emotional flexibility, and a wellness safety net.

Burnout and triggers

Burnout includes work-related stress, emotional and physical exhaustion, depersonalization, decreased motivation, decreased personal accomplishment, and reduced performance. Causes of burnout include time pressures, chaotic environments, low control of pace, EHR interactions, and non-work stressors like family responsibilities.[1] There are organizational, systemic, and personal factors that lead to burnout. Burnout also has the potential to manifest as mental health concerns and suicidal ideation.

Physician burnout rose during the pandemic, which was coupled with increases in emotional exhaustion and depersonalization. The rise in burnout likely drove career changes among physicians during this time period.[2] As an example of increasing stressors, health care provider inboxes from patient portal messages at the University of Chicago grew in volume nearly 235 percent during the pandemic (2020-2021).

Burnout may carry an increased risk of emotional distress, depression, substance use, and suicidal ideation. Physicians and nurses are at higher risk of suicide than the general population.[2,3] The relative risk of suicide for female physicians is 2.27, and 1.41, for males compared to the general population.[2] Physicians in training experience a 370 percent increase in suicidal ideation.[2]

An area of focus to combat burnout is EHR optimization including patient messaging innovation, streamlining physician workflow, decreasing mental load, improving the experience of the EHR,[2] and "getting rid of stupid stuff."[2] The application of AI in areas like ambient documentation and patient message responses also can serve to improve interactions with the EHR.

#WhatToFix

#WhatToFix is an initiative to crowdsource problems and solutions, known colloquially and humorously as #WTF. The purpose of #WTF is to provide a single point of contact for providers and teams to advance fixable challenges for prioritization and resolution, and in doing so, empower clinical staff and reduce helplessness and burnout. #WTF uses a fix framework that utilizes purpose, infrastructure and capacity, defined process, recent fixes, and crowdsourcing and communication.

The ideal scope for a #WTF problem is any small fix that will improve the ease of clinical practice or reduce daily frustrations. Any clinician across the system can request a fix. The submission form includes the questions: "What is the problem that you would like to be fixed?" and "What is your anticipated solution to the problem?"Requesters are referred to the IT Help line to address immediate concerns such as usernames, passwords, or E-mail. EHR break/fix issues are out of scope. The program has expanded to include non-informatics requests addressing facilities, operations, and other concerns.

The #WTF team leverages the health informatics team. Fixes are prioritized based on clinical context and the understanding of clinical workflows. The #WTF program sets an expectation that there will be timely review and triage of issues. It can be integrated with a service ticket platform that is viewable to submitters which allows for transparency and tracking on a dashboard of submissions. Submitters are notified when a fix is routed to another team or solved. The program maintains a resource list with one to two point persons identified across the domains of potential issues. The goal is to get fixes to the correct person in the correct operational or clinical area.

The core team for #WTF consists of a program manager, health informaticists, and clinical informatics fellows. Leadership includes the Chief Medical Officer, Chief Wellness and Vitality Officer. Fulfillment teams include informatics, information technology, facilities, parking, human resources, and operational teams. This larger team also serves to escalate issues, identify larger opportunities, link fixes to ongoing work, and flag and share successes. The technology involved includes the service ticket platform, the EHR, E-mail and reporting tools.

Fixes fall into four phenotypes, a fix that can be directed to an EHR builder and corrected almost straight away; a fix that uses multiple services and processes to improve; a fix that is larger in scope but significant at the organizational level for future prioritization; or a fix that is not quite a possibility or probability in the near future.

A #WhatToFix highlight newsletter is sent on a monthly basis via E-mail outlining recent fixes and other important updates. It sometimes includes tip sheets or special reminders regarding new processes in the EHR. It also emphasizes gratitude for clinicians taking time to connect with the #WTF team.

From 2017-2023 500 total fixes were submitted. Of these, 75 percent were EHR and IT related, and 25 percent operations or facilities related. The team addressed 85 percent of fixes, leaving 15 percent of the fixes out of current scope or low priority. Recent examples of fixes include improving the reporting view for blood transfusions; allowing language interpretation through an app on personal devices; including commonly used clinical documents in the mobile EHR application; organizing 24 hour labs in a panel; newborn alert for bilirubin testing based on hours; and an alert offering a naloxone prescription to go with narcotic prescriptions.

In 2023, the #WTF team received 52 submissions, and were able to address 25 of these. Highlights from the year include increasing the login timeout for EHR; adding a 48-hour result smart link; clinical document scanning workflow redesign; room number displays in mobile EHR applications; and improving parking flow and understanding.

Changing culture is critical

Embracing the culture of well-being is critical at the organizational level. Practically, changing culture can take many forms. Fixing systems that are easy to access and that respond to clinician input is one mechanism to improve culture. Furthermore, the communication of successes has been a way to share one person's fix, broadly, as often hundreds of clinicians want similar solutions.

References

1. StanfordMedicine . WellMD & WellPhD. The Stanford Model of Professional Fulfillment™. https://wellmd.stanford.edu/about/model-external.html last accessed 1/18/24.
2. Agency for Healthcare Research and Quality. Physician Burnout. https://www.ahrq.gov/prevention/clinician/ahrq-works/burnout/index.html.
3. Shanafelt, T, et al. Changes in Burnout and Satisfaction With Work-Life Integration in Physicians During the First 2 Years of the COVID-19 Pandemic. Mayo Clinic Proc. Dec, 97(12): 2248-58.
4. Saley, C. Survey: Nearly half of physicians changed jobs during the pandemic. CHG Healthcare. 27 Jun. 2022. https://chghealthcare.com/blog/physicians-changed-jobs-survey#:~:text=A%20 2022%20CHG%20Healthcare%20survey,physicians%20is%206%2D7%25.
5. Davis MA, Cher BAY, Friese CR, Bynum JPW. Association of US Nurse and Physician Occupation With Risk of Suicide. JAMA Psychiatry. 2021 Apr 14; 78(6): 1–8.
6. Dyrbye LN, Thomas MR, Massie FS, Power DV, Eacker A, Harper W, Durning S, Moutier C, Szydlo DW, Novotny PJ, Sloan JA, Shanafelt TD. Burnout and suicidal ideation among U.S. medical students. Ann Intern Med. 2008 Sep 2; 149(5): 334-41.
7. Schernhammer ES, Colditz GA. Suicide rates among physicians: a quantitative and gender assessment (meta-analysis). Am J Psychiatry. 2004 Dec; 161(12): 2295-302. .
8. Sen S, Kranzler HR, Krystal JH, Speller H, Chan G, Gelernter J, Guille C. A prospective cohort study investigating factors associated with depression during medical internship. Arch Gen Psychiatry. 2010 Jun; 67(6): 557-65.
9. Strudwick G, Jeffs L, Kemp J, Sequeira L, Lo B, Shen N, Paterson P, Coombe N, Yang L, Ronald K, Wang W, Pagliaroli S, Tajirian T, Ling S, Jankowicz D. Identifying and adapting interventions to reduce documentation burden and improve nurses' efficiency in using electronic health record systems (The IDEA Study): protocol for a mixed methods study. BMC Nurs. 2022 Aug 4; 21(1): 213.
10. Ashton M. Getting Rid of Stupid Stuff. N Engl J Med. 2018 Nov 8; 379(19): 1789-91.

Chapter 12

The future of care delivery

Vin Gupta, MD, MPA

Can artificial intelligence make you healthier? Can you tell if your heart is failing by going to the bathroom? Will a fungus cause our next pandemic?

There is immense opportunity to improve access to health care through current technologies. One example is a toilet with sensors to monitor a person's pulse, blood pressure, and oxygen levels while sitting on the toilet as part of their daily routine. Another is a mirror that looks into your eyes while you brush your teeth and retrieves your vital signs.

In addition, data collection improvements from smartwatches could prove more effective than blood pressure cuffs because more people wear smartwatches and the data is more reliable.

New blood tests for specific T-cells to screen for cancers can be more accurate and cost-effective than a whole-body MRI, or the current one-cancer-specific tests like colonoscopies or mammograms.

Artificial intelligence is part of health care and shouldn't be feared. AI is helping in medical record-keeping so doctors can spend more time with patients. It sorts through massive amounts of data to help make predictive diagnoses that doctors can then take under advisement. It reviews patient data, identifies gaps, and can help providers target care patients may be missing. This is the next generation of WebMD, but with more personalized answers.

Even with AI, a shortage looms

The most urgent threat to our health isn't a microscopic virus or strain of bacteria. It's a shortage of doctors. More than 83 million Americans don't have sufficient access to a primary care provider.[1] Within a decade, the United States could be short almost 50,000 primary care physicians.[2]

Educating and training more doctors is critical, but will take years, even decades. In the meantime, we need to maximize the capacity of our existing corps of providers by making the health system more efficient and managing illness more proactively.

In other words, we have to learn how to do more with less. An ongoing revolution in digital health care delivery—from telehealth visits to pharmacies that deliver to the home—can help do just that.

However, first, a reality check. The health care status quo isn't working for most patients. Seven in 10 Americans say the system isn't meeting their needs, according to data from a 2023 Harris Poll.[3]

Wait times are the top concern. As a physician, I've seen firsthand how our system forces patients to wait weeks for care, even for the most routine and easily treatable health conditions. New patients wait 26 days,[4] on average, to see a primary care physician.

On the day of the appointment, the average patient waits nearly 20 minutes to see their provider for a 20-minute appointment.

Delays in care aren't just inconvenient, they have real-world consequences for patient health and the broader economy. Seeing a primary care doctor can prevent a manageable health issue from evolving into a life-threatening illness.

Optimizing health care

Telemedicine can help to bring efficiency to the sluggish status quo. Virtual appointments optimize doctors' time, allowing providers to see and triage more patients in a day. And, virtually treating patients with routine health conditions can free up capacity at emergency rooms and other facilities focused on in-person care.

Patients benefit, too. Telemedicine eliminates the need to travel and can reduce how long patients have to wait for care. It's no surprise that virtual appointments are associated with fewer last-minute cancellations, which can sap a physician's productivity.

But how do we reconcile telemedicine with the continued need for in-person diagnostics and lab work?

Integrating virtual care with remote patient-monitoring tools can help providers receive real-time updates on their patients' blood glucose, blood pressure, and more. It allows doctors to better monitor, communicate with, and prescribe medicines for patients.

Remote patient-monitoring tools can also help with ensuring patients can take the medicines their doctors prescribe, which also will boost the health system's productivity. Too often, patients don't or are unable to adhere to recommended treatment regimens, which can allow manageable conditions to snowball into life-threatening emergencies.

Millions of Americans land in the hospital each year because of chronic conditions, which affect an estimated six in 10 Americans.[5] For diabetes and high blood pressure, medication adherence rates are typically at 50 percent to 60 percent of prescribed doses.[6] Nonadherence results in more than $300 billion in avoidable health care costs[7] in the U.S. every year.[7] About 125,000 Americans die[8] annually because of nonadherence.[8]

Making it easier for patients to take their medicines as directed with online alternatives to traditional pharmacies can help solve this crisis. One study of Medicare Part D patients with chronic conditions found that those who used pharmacy delivery services were significantly more likely to adhere to their prescriptions.[9] Consumers who hesitate to use mail-order pharmacy services are most concerned about delivery speed and a perceived lack of personal connection. Fortunately, several companies are working to address these potential roadblocks by delivering drugs faster, and offering more personalized care.

Patients are also discouraged from sticking to their medication regimen when they pick up their medications at the pharmacy only to find out that the cost is more than expected, and often unaffordable. Online alternatives often make prices clear upfront, and sometimes are less expensive than going through insurance.[10]

Better adoption of new technologies such as AI, telemedicine, and pharmacy delivery can streamline the health care experience for patients and physicians alike, and help providers who are stretched thin to triage care and better ensure the health of their patients. It's time for the U.S. health care system to adopt these continuously developing new technologies and meet patients where they are.

References

1. American Medical Association. AMA president sounds alarm on national physician shortage. October 25, 2034. https://www.ama-assn.org/press-center/press-releases/ama-president-sounds-alarm-national-physician-shortage.
2. Fleron A, Singhal S. The gathering storm: The uncertain future of US healthcare. McKinsey & Company. September 16, 2022. https://www.mckinsey.com/industries/healthcare/our-insights/the-gathering-storm-the-uncertain-future-of-us-healthcare.
3. American Academy of Physician Associates. The Harris Poll. The Patient Experience: Perspective on Today's Healthcare. https://www.aapa.org/research/patient-experience/.
4. Levine H. How to get in to see primary care physicians and specialists – quickly: The average wait for an appointment with a physician for new patients is 26 days, according to a 2022 survey of 15 metropolitan areas. The Washington Post. Consumer Reports. October 30, 2023. https://www.washingtonpost.com/wellness/2023/10/30/medical-appointments-avoiding-long-waits/.
5. Centers for Disease Control. Chronic Disease. https://www.cdc.gov/chronic-disease/#:~:text=Six percent20in percent20ten percent20Americans percent20live,driver percent20of percent20health percent20care percent20costs.
6. Sahoo J, Mohanty S, Kundu A, Epari V. Medication Adherence Among Patients of Type II Diabetes Mellitus and Its Associated Risk Factors: A Cross-Sectional Study in A Tertiary Care Hospital of Eastern India. Cureus. 2022 Dec; 14(12): e33074.

7. Car J, Tan WS, Huang Z, Sloot P, Franklin BD. eHealth in the future of medications management: personalisation, monitoring and adherence. BMC Med. 2017; 15: 73.
8. Benhamin RM. Medication Adherence: Helping Patients Take Their Medicines As Directed. Public Health Rep. 2012 Jan-Feb; 127(1): 2-3.
9. Iyengar RN, LeFrancois AL, Henderson RR, Rabbitt RM. Medication Nonadherence Among Medicare Beneficiaries with Comorbid Chronic Conditions: Influence of Pharmacy Dispensing Channel. J Manag Care Spec Pharm. 2016 May; 22(5): 10.
10. Lovelace Jr B. Online pharmacy programs can save patients millions in prescription drug costs, study finds. NBC News: Health News. September 4, 2023. https://www.nbcnews.com/health/health-news/online-pharmacy-programs-can-patients-millions-prescription-drug-costs-rcna102783.

Concluding remarks

Upholding professionalism in a transformative era of medicine

Bradley E. Barth, MD, MSLOD;
Oluwaferanmi O. Okanlami, MD, MS; and Juan N. Lessing, MD, FACP

In the spirit of the 2023 AOA conference upon which this monograph was conceived—"Professionalism in a Relentless World"—which unsurprisingly drew heavily on the opportunity and peril of technology, we have opted to try our hand writing this conclusion with the aid of large language model (LLM) artificial intelligence (AI), specifically OpenAI's ChatGPT, version ChatGPT 4 Turbo. We started by asking ChatGPT to find the common threads that tie all the preceding chapters together and to weave a cohesive summary. We have made edits, corrections, and rewrites where we felt the technology fell short. Human expertise, or at least experience, we feel, remains critical. We conclude our conclusion with a reflection on the use of this technology as a writing aid. Below is the amalgam of machine and human.[1]

In today's complex healthcare landscape, medical professionalism continues to serve as the foundation of effective and ethical care. This monograph has explored the multidimensional challenges and opportunities of professionalism in medicine, offering diverse perspectives on how the field can evolve while holding fast to its core values of compassion, integrity, and patient-centered care. This conclusion synthesizes key insights from each chapter, illustrating how medicine can thrive through thoughtful adaptation, collaborative practice, and a commitment to lifelong learning.

The monograph opens with Dr. Richard Byyny's exploration of communities of practice and the enduring value of face-to-face communication in medical education and practice. He highlights how in-person learning fosters mentorship, shared experiences, and collaboration that no technological tool can replicate. This foundation is complemented by the work of Drs. Molly Jackson and David Hatem, who address the challenges of connection and community in an increasingly digital era

1-Prompt: Please read through this PDF and create a final chapter that is a concluding chapter that summarizes all of the other chapters and brings everything together nicely.
-Prompt: Could you please provide another version of this, pulling examples from the chapters themselves as well?"
-Prompt: We asked ChatGPT to write a conclusion for a monograph for the alpha omega alpha medical honor society for a conference that took place. I will copy and paste what chatgpt wrote. Then I will attach the monograph on what this conclusion is supposed to be based. I then want to ask you several questions and requests.
-Prompt: Does the conclusion talk about every chapter/submission (I think there are 12) or only some?
-Prompt: Analyze more thoroughly. [ChatGPT came back saying it had omitted Chapters 8, 9, and 10]
-Prompt: Revise the conclusion to address the missing chapters. It would be strange to mention all but a few chapters. That seems insulting.
-Prompt: is it correct to call our monograph based from a conference too have been born from it? that sounds weird
-Prompt: Help me revise this sentence to not use "digestible" in order to avoid mixed metaphors: We started by asking ChatGPT to find the common threads that tie all the preceding chapters together and to weave a digestible summary.
-Prompt: list your chatgpt version. How would I reference you

of medical education. They advocate for intentional strategies, such as longitudinal mentorship and collaborative learning, to prevent isolation and promote professional identity formation (PIF) among trainees.

Dr. Olaoluwa Fayanju reflects on the evolution of medical professionalism, emphasizing that while the principles of beneficence, non-maleficence, and confidentiality remain timeless, they require reinterpretation to address modern challenges like data privacy and the ethical use of technologies to ensure they improve health outcomes, not exacerbate existing disparities, and avoid unanticipated new problems. Expanding on this theme, Dr. Steven Wartman explores AI in healthcare, reminding us that while AI holds great promise in diagnostics and efficiency, its integration must be tempered by ethical vigilance, transparency, and the irreplaceable value of human judgment.

Dr. Marie Sandoval examines the impact of digital tools on patient connections, stressing the importance of maintaining empathy and trust in virtual interactions. Similarly, Dr. Eve Higginbotham and colleagues advocate for inclusive leadership as a transformative model for healthcare organizations, illustrating how diversity and equity strengthen the profession and foster innovation.

Drs. Douglas Paauw and Jenny Wright explore the benefits of OpenNotes in clinical documentation, outlining both the potential to enhance trust and the complexities of navigating transparency with sensitivity. Dr. Jay Brahmbhatt sheds light on the hypocrisy that can arise in the clinical learning environment, calling for an honest reassessment of institutional practices that may undermine professional ideals, such as disparities in treatment and systemic inequities.

Drs. Lynn Buckvar-Keltz and Barbara Porter turn their attention to supporting professional identity formation in medical trainees. They emphasize the critical role of socialization, reflection, and mentorship in cultivating a physician's sense of belonging and purpose, particularly in the face of societal and professional pressures. Building on this, Dr. Antoinette Pusateri and colleagues examine medical professionalism in an evolving landscape, offering a nuanced perspective on how physicians can adapt to rapid changes in healthcare while preserving the values that anchor the profession.

Addressing the well-being of clinicians, Dr. Bryan Hendrickson and colleagues highlight strategies to combat burnout through innovative technology and systemic support. Finally, Dr. Vin Gupta envisions the future of care delivery in an era of transformation, advocating for a systems-oriented approach to improve both physician well-being and patient outcomes.

Taken together, these chapters underscore that professionalism in medicine today is defined by a delicate balance: preserving time-honored values while embracing innovation and inclusivity. Professionalism requires that physicians not only master clinical knowledge but also uphold ethical standards, nurture human connections, and lead with integrity and resilience. By fostering a culture of reflection, collaboration, and equity, the medical profession can remain a source of trust and inspiration in a rapidly evolving world. In the spirit of the Alpha Omega Alpha Honor Medical Society's enduring mission to "be worthy to serve the suffering," this monograph concludes with a renewed commitment to advancing professionalism as the cornerstone of medicine.

Reflections on writing with AI

AI does a surprisingly good job, albeit superficially, of summarizing large amounts of data. Skimmed, what ChatGPT produced sounds convincing. However, several glaring deficiencies shined through. The first iterations missed several chapters/authors. We had to ask and double check three times to ensure no one was skipped. Perhaps by necessity, the first pass was, just that, a superficial pass. Perhaps it is not fair to ask that a one or two-sentence summary capture deep sentiment. But isn't that the task of a concluding chapter or summary, the role of the editors, and the beauty (and pain) of skilled writing? Editing, writing and rewriting the conclusion still required close reading, contextual understanding, and choices. Luckily for authors everywhere, just as much for physicians, this experience and this monograph that the human endeavor of writing and medicine very much still requires and benefits from human practitioners.